Ghostwoman:

The Mystical Experience of a Housewife/Physician

An Unconditional Love Story

In gratitude for your interest & support. Blessings on the journey,
♡ *Harriet*

Ghostwoman:

The Mystical Experience of a Housewife/Physician

An Unconditional Love Story

Harriet Cohen, M.D.

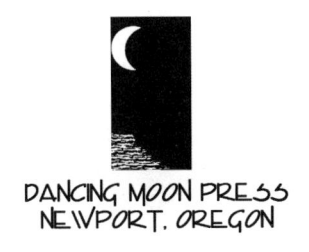

DANCING MOON PRESS
NEWPORT, OREGON

Ghostwoman

© 2005 by Harriet Cohen, MD

ALL RIGHTS RESERVED

No part of this book may be reproduced or transmitted in any form, by any means, without written permission from the author.

Published by DANCING MOON PRESS
P.O. Box 832, Newport, OR 97365
Printed in the United States of America

Book Design: Carla Perry
Cover art and design: Karen Downs
Printed by: McNaughton-Gunn
Manufactured in the United States of America

Library of Congress Control Number: 2005922507
ISBN: 1-892076-15-2
Cohen, Harriet, MD,
Ghostwoman
1. Title; 2. Memoir;
3. Spirituality; 4. Psychology

FIRST EDITION

Contents

Acknowledgements ii
Preface vi

PART I

1 Pathfinder 17
2 Descent 29
3 Healing Begins 54
4 The Next Three Months 60
5 Of God and Madness 77
6 On Being, Madness? and Creating A Mess 91
7 Settling Down 114
8 Evaluation #1 131
9 The Reports 143
10 Rolling up My Sleeves 159

PART II

11 Validation 183
12 Diagnosis #2 201
13 New Demands 212
14 Four More Opinions 226
15 The Hearing 249
16 First Response 272
17 Rage 287
18 Unconditional Love 305
19 Loose Ends 325
    Epilogue 341
    Bibliography & Recommended Reading 343

Acknowledgments

It is with deepest appreciation to the following people, that the writing of this book was made possible:

First, to my husband, without whose strength of spirit I could not have come to know my own. Not only were you a huge piece of the inspiration for this book, you have financially supported us through a large part of my writing it, even when you had a hard time with what I was writing.

To my children, whose independence, patience, and happiness gave me the time I needed to focus on this work for long stretches of time. You are precious beyond words, and a great joy to me when I come up for air.

To my parents, both by birth and by marriage, who have inspired me to look deeply into the meaning of all things, and taught me different faces of love by your examples.

To Carolyn Altman, who suffered through my first few drafts and took my earliest, single-spaced writing seriously. You are a great teacher, and without your emotional clarity, I might never have begun to understand this period of my life as deeply as I have. Too bad I had to cut the scene with you swatting those flies. Love that memory! But as you taught me to ask, it didn't exactly serve the story.

To my early readers: Paula, Cindy, Sheera, Nancy, Gretta, Carolyn, Robin, Kirsten, Dorothy, and Karen, thank you for being such kind and gentle souls. I needed just that to have the courage to ask for feedback for such a personal piece of work. Your gentleness was much appreciated, as much as the fact that you liked my writing. You make a great team of editors!

To Carol Adler, for giving my earlier version a serious look, and considering my book for publication. Having a publisher who was interested kept me going when I was ready to be done with this and to move on with my life. Your insights and suggestions were invaluable. Thanks for not accepting *Ghostwoman* in her initial naked form. It allowed me the time to highlight what was needed, and modestly veil those parts that would have led to unnecessary discomfort for myself and others.

To my friends at the Old Wholeness Center, for confirming my sanity and connecting me to vital resources that knew the difference. Thank you for your courage to make your own lives genuine, and creating such a welcoming community.

To the Institute of Noetic Science, and The American Holistic Medical Association, for your reverence for the marriage between science and spirituality. And deepest thanks to our local chapters for reaching out and finding me. Your ongoing support, love, and our regular meetings keep reminding me that I still belong.

To Dr. Bice and Dr. Paltrow for your wonderful support, and for your courage to speak out your truth in opposition to the system. You helped me to not to take those other voices too seriously.

To Thomas McDermott and Ted Runstein, for being wonderful lawyers and people, making me much less cynical about the legal profession. Hope you are right about me being able to publish this stuff, Thomas!

To all the teachers who took the time to write their wisdom down for me: Dr. Caroline Myss; David Simon, MD; Deepak Chopra MD; Brian Weiss, MD; Stanislav Grof, MD; Larry Dossey MD; Dennis Gersten, MD, Dr. Paula Kaplan, and Dr. Abraham Maslow. You began my journey of studying from a deep place of passion. Thank you for finding the time to write so eloquently and understandably.

To Dr. Eugene K. for your narrow minded understanding of my experience. Had you not assessed me as you did, I would not have had much of a story to write, nor would I have had time to process all these things or do very much of my studying. Thanks for the break!

To Betsy Charleston, whose personal integrity and compassion for patients and personnel has always been a gift to the world. Your perspective of my experience was instrumental in my moving on. You were the mama bird kicking this baby bird out of the nest in which I no longer fit. It was time for me to learn to spread my own wings, whether I make it or not. And thank you for your continued support and words of encouragement after all these years.

To Mrs. Bloom, for whatever happened in your car. This was a necessary event to allow my shell to crack open. The pain in my leg is nothing compared to the joy in my heart, and I would never have known the latter without the former.

To that separate consciousness that came into my body for two short weeks. Some relationships are not meant to live out their potential at a particular time. You have always been loved. You will always be loved. And we will meet again when the stars are so aligned and the moon fills the sky with brilliance.

To Rabbi Avram, who teaches me much about Judaism, and through that, much about myself. Your passion for our story, our people, and all people, is precious. May we each be a light for the other.

To Rabbi Ariyeh, for helping me with my last ethical question about publishing my story, and being the sort of person I could ask to read my manuscript.

To Karen and Carla, my midwives, for finally delivering this creation. I couldn't have done it without you.

Lastly, my wholehearted appreciation to God. For being such a mystery, and such a Love. Thanks for creating us to find each other. Thanks for the opportunity to become conscious.

Preface

"Every truth we see is ours to give the world, not to keep for ourselves alone, for in so doing we cheat humanity out of their rights, and check our own development." -
Elizabeth Cady Stanton

As I wind down and into the last two chapters of the twelfth draft of *Ghostwoman*, I find myself surrounded by sunlight, rainbow prisms on the wall, tears and fears, pain and clarity. I am coming down the home stretch, distracted by the fleeting thoughts that come to me about this six-year process I have undergone. With each draft, not only did the manuscript of *Ghostwoman* change, but ghostwoman changed as well.

Six years of a cocoon, often grieving to be back in the world in some more productive way. But it wasn't time yet. This last draft feels like time. Finally, I understand this book I have been writing, this book that has been writing me.

i am, this, i am.

Ghostwoman is a story about a relationship with God. It is written, and lived, through the eyes of a forty-one-year-old mother and half-time physician who has lost herself in her work as a mother, wife, and physician. This loss of ego is not an exalted state of oneness with the world, but rather a broken state of being in the world with no desire for being at all. To lose one's ego is to lose one's greatest gift, the gift of our unique being and meaning. It is what no one but ourselves can bring to this wholeness we call life, and to lose ourselves is one of the most devastating losses we can endure.

This was ghostwoman.

Her story is one of self-discovery, and as part of that journey, the discovery of the Self, through an extraordinary experience of mystical consciousness. Here, ghostwoman not only discovers her personal relationship with God and the importance of herself in that relationship, but she experiences the deepest, most unconditional love — the essence of all things.

She returns from her experience as a defender of wholeness in a world where brokenness is the norm. Her life becomes the canvas upon which she learns how to paint this picture of unconditional love, where she begins to understand its complicated yet simple expression in this world, and where she deepens her understanding of her relationship with the *One* that is her teacher.

Ego and egolessness; the dance of co-creation that makes life eternal.

Ghostwoman is a memoir, and as such it is true to my memory of these events. Most of the events were written as they happened, and I've included some journal entries to reflect the truth of those days in the language and sentiment of that time. I also sent the portions that included others to many of the individuals, to ask whether I had misrepresented any of our shared experiences. On only one account was there a question. I had remembered someone saying something they did not remember saying, and they felt the words were out of their character. Although I thought I remembered it clearly, I know well enough that memory is a perfectly imperfect resource, and so I chose to make the statement a generic one, rather than one said by the individual. This is the only time that I compromised my retelling of this story, though I did choose to delete portions that put others in an unfavorable light unless those situations were critical to the point of the story.

I have also changed the names of many of the individuals in an effort to help them maintain a bit of privacy. The exposure of writing a memoir is not one that we all are ready for, and I hope my effort is helpful in limiting discomfort for others. My apologies to those whose identities are not so easily concealed.

The purpose of this memoir has not been to humiliate anyone, but rather to use these events to highlight a way to walk through life with God, and with love.

Unconditional Love is founded in truth. And it is to truth that this memoir is devoted. May *Ghostwoman* inspire each of us to claim our own truths; to love ourselves in spite of them and because of them, and to grow from them because we claim the courage to become aware and choose to be something different than we've been. More honest and whole, more in love with ourselves and each other.

May our love expand exponentially in this truth! And may it be the source of all healing, great joy, and deep peace.

Ghostwoman:

The Mystical Experience of a Housewife/Physician

An Unconditional Love Story

Within the mundane
lies the seed of the extraordinary
waiting
for the moment of perfection
when the shell splits apart
and surprise bursts forth
that is newer than imaginable
and as old as the beginning.
A room full of colors
explodes from invisible white light
shot through a prism.
The colors were always there.

Part I

Chapter 1
Path Finder

It is hard to say how I felt that October Third afternoon. To say I was weak is an understatement. I was beyond weak, I was a ghostwoman. My long thin legs ended in nothingness. They carried me from place to place, as they were commanded. My arms did as they were told, they held the 'For Sale By Owner' sign vertical while my husband filled the deep hole he had just dug in the rocky flowerbed. My belly was a plate of armor.

The sun streamed brightly down as I helped Frank plant the sign. Cool, autumn air kept me from sweating. The dahlias were still blooming off to the right, but the rose bushes beside me displayed only thorns. They had given up their summer blooming and the leaves had fallen to black spot in our organic flower garden by the edge of the two-lane highway.

A stream of cars whooshed by along the busy road, leaving behind a cloud of foul smelling air. I didn't even try to hold my breath until the dusty exhaust cleared a bit, as I was usually inspired to do. I breathed it in, not caring.

"It looks straight to me," I said flatly. The street was temporarily quiet, so I didn't have to raise my voice to be heard above the din of the traffic.

Ghostwoman

I looked at my watch. 2:35 pm. I had just enough time to walk to the bakery, pick up the bread, and come home before picking up my son Jade from school. It would be tight. If I drove to the bakery I wouldn't be quite so rushed. But we lived so close that I couldn't drive without feeling guilty for adding all that pollution for such a minuscule errand. Besides, it might take me just as long to find a parking space as it would to walk. If I hurried I had time.

Impatiently, I waited for the long line of vehicles to stop streaming by. They'd pause in one direction, only to start zooming in the other. Finally a break allowed me to jog across between cars. A drainage ditch was next to me, too wide to hop across to the narrow dirt path on the other side. Long quick strides moved my feet along the edge of the river of asphalt.

I waved to the newsstand-coffee shop owner as I passed by. They'd added a nice touch to the neighborhood when they fixed up that ugly old building. I'd miss saying hello, but not miss feeling bad about giving them so little business. I didn't drink coffee anymore and I didn't have time to read the magazines that came to the house, let alone buy more. The kids liked the candy and cocoa with fresh whipped cream, but the street was too busy for them to cross alone, and I was too busy to walk them, and there was cocoa in our cabinets.

I stepped into the bakery, glancing at the clock, then at the two women in front of me. One had an infant, the other a toddler. The toddler, a little boy with curly blond hair, huge eyes, and thick lashes, was dressed in long pants and suspenders. Running back and forth along the glass cases looking at all the colorful pastries and the plastic birthday cake decorations, he reminded me of Jade when he was that age, about seven years ago. He, too, had worn suspenders – red ones, and climbed on the little shelf, which was supposed to be for handbags. The boy and his mother were as oblivious to the 'Do Not Climb On

Chapter 1: Path Finder

Shelf' sign as Jade and I had once been.

It was all I could do to keep my eyes on him, there was no time for reading signs.

I felt a tightness in my throat and a heaviness in my chest, as I shifted my attention to the infant. It lay nestled in the sling, too close to its mother for me to get much of a look at. I could feel it as if it hung on my own body in front of my heart. A soft head popped out of the top. How I'd loved to caress the smooth, warm heads of my own babies. They'd fit into the palm of my hand so perfectly. My fingers would softly massage, revel in the touch of something so warm and smooth and alive. So perfect. I remembered turning my hand so that I could stroke their satiny cheeks with the less calloused side of my fingers.

The moms finished with their selections and moved off to sit at the small round table at the other side of the little bakery. The mother of the toddler called him over from the bakery case. He was having so much fun eying the goodies that he had forgotten he had his own waiting at the table. He turned and ran back to her.

"Hi, Mrs. Cohen. Would you like anything besides your challah?"

I'd been buying the braided Jewish egg bread from this bakery every Friday for Shabbat, since we moved into the neighborhood. It was one of the handful of rituals from my Judaism that had meaning for me. One day of rest a week. What a perfect commandment! And though it had no practical significance for a working mother, it was a beautiful ideal that I at least enjoyed for the evening. If not a full day of rest, at least a conscious pause to praise, and appreciate, and to look for the meaning in all things.

We sang three blessings every week, to welcome Shabbat. The first, as we lit Shabbat candles, was for light. For understanding and wisdom. The second we sang as we raised glasses filled with wine or grape juice. It was a praise over the fruit of the vine, that which is made purely by the creator. The last, the braided bread, was in my

Ghostwoman

mind a symbol of how the past, present, and future are all woven together, a symbol of our co-creation with God.

The bakery had called a week before to remind me of the upcoming High Holidays. "Would you like the usual braided loaf, or the round turban challah? With or without raisins?"

The round loaf, a reminder of the circular nature of all things. Raisins, a symbol for a sweet new year. I'd have forgotten these things without the reminder from my Japanese and German bakers.

I glanced around briefly, my eyes falling on the day-old turban challahs for a buck cheaper. We were four days into having two mortgages.

"Could I buy the day-old challah instead?" I asked with embarrassment.

And was answered with an explosion.

Glass shattered everywhere and my eyes instinctively clamped shut as I curled into a ball.

Had a bomb been planted in the bakery because it was selling Jewish bread? I'd read about such stories all my life.

I opened my eyes and found myself suspended above the floor, my knees squeezed tightly together and bent as if I were sitting in a chair with my legs tucked underneath. I was pinned sideways between the glass display counter and a large vehicle, a Pathfinder, which had smoke streaming from the engine. My legs felt crushed, but I didn't feel much pain right away.

A pedestrian outside was yelling for a fire extinguisher.

I glanced up at the clock. 3:00 pm. Iyra, my daughter, would be getting dropped off at home about now and it was time to pick up Jade from school.

Was the smoking car about to explode and engulf me in flames? Would I ever see Jade and Iyra again?

With the thought of my children's sadness if I were to die an untimely death, I attempted to wriggle free. That

Chapter 1: Path Finder

was when the searing pain filled my legs as I tried to lift my right leg up, to free it from the cold embrace of the steel. My right foot was no longer well attached to my leg, but was somehow dangling from my lower shin. I gave up trying to move.

Gudrun, one of the owners, came out from the back. Her eyes doubled in size as her gaze landed on my pinned body. "Are you OK?!"

"No, my leg's broken," I answered calmly.

Then I added, with a bit more urgency, "Call 911. And then, could you call my husband? He's at home, painting the house."

Gudrun disappeared into the back.

I watched the scene around me. The watchers and the movers, like little ants milling about on the other side of where the windows had been. Someone was climbing through the opening that was framed in shattered glass. Someone was trying to talk to the driver. I couldn't see her, but I heard voices saying she seemed unhurt, but stunned or something.

Barry came out from the back. His gentle, Japanese eyes braced and widened with concern. "No one is answering. I left a message."

"My husband's there, I know he is. He's painting the house. We live just up the road. We're the fifth house on the right after the overpass. There's a "For Sale" sign out in front. Could someone please just go and get him?"

The acrid smell of burnt rubber and smoldering plastic mingled with the exhaust and the aroma of sugar, almond paste and berries. Sirens were coming closer. If I didn't move my legs, if I kept my breathing above my waist, I hardly felt the pain.

Barry tried the phone again. Frank answered, having just caught enough of the first message to hear that his wife was pinned by a car in some store. He raced up the street, leaving the house wide open, and was at my side by the time the paramedics began extricating me onto the top of the counter. Despite their trying to handle the pieces of my broken limb carefully, the sharp edges of bones grated against each other as I was moved. Frank held my hand while I squeezed his, taking the edge off the pain. Someone brought out a bag of ice and put it on my deformed leg.

"I deserved this," I whispered, my chest tightening and my eyes welling with tears.

"No you didn't," Frank responded softly. But I wasn't listening. I looked away. If I looked at him, it would all come pouring out. So I swallowed my tears in the tightness of my throat that almost strangled me.

"You need to get home," I finally was able to say.

"Iyra's probably been dropped off already, and Jade's waiting at school. Pick him up with Iyra and you can meet me at the emergency room." I managed a smile. "I'll be OK."

But he did not leave my side until I was out of the bakery. We held hands as he walked with me and my paramedic entourage through the back of the shop, past the crumbling wall with the falling shelves, the sink that had become dislocated from the wall, past the mist that filled the air from the broken water pipe, past the sympathetic faces of my bakers, and the dust of destruction that would linger long after the broken body had moved on.

Do you know what a ghostwoman is?

She is a woman who has lived so much for others that she rarely inhabits her own body. She smiles regularly, but it's the smile that is a gift, not an expression of her personal feelings. A ghostwoman doesn't know how she feels. At some point, she doesn't even know what she thinks.

Oh, she has opinions. But they are safe things that she is talking about, nothing that would dramatically threaten the status quo of her life. Ghostwomen don't

Chapter 1: Path Finder

have the flesh they need to go to the edge, explore, and quite possibly to make a mistake.

Making a decision is one of the most difficult things for a ghostwoman, because although she is making the decision, it is rarely her decision she ends up making.

That was me in those days, as self-assured as I appeared to others.

I'd lost touch with who I was, particularly with the parts of me that thrived on life. I couldn't remember the last time I'd laughed a deep soulful laugh, and it was rare for me to play so that I felt alive and filled with joy. I remembered kindness and generosity, but I didn't feel them. And I'd long forgotten how much fun I once had contemplating the nature of God, despite my old irreverence at religious school.

The worst part was that I didn't even know I'd forgotten all these things. That is the way of forgetting. All I knew was how to get through the day. How to put one foot in front of the next one with a smile on my face and a kind word whenever possible. How to go through the motions. How to make lists so I wouldn't forget one of the many details that controlled my life. But it was rare anymore for me to feel things in my heart .

I was an ordinary woman, and had an ordinary life of mother, wife, and half-time physician. I grew up with four brothers and two parents in the suburbs of South Florida. Was a good student, but had to work at it. Stayed out of trouble. Got three Ouija boards one birthday and could never get any of them to move. Didn't have premonitions, see auras, and rarely had a dream that made much sense. Only once, as a child, did I have *deja vu*.

But within six months I would have a mystical experience that would begin to unravel the tapestry of the life I'd been creating. The threads would come apart, at first by force, later by choice. It was as if my precious spun fibers needed to be freed for a creation that was far more expressive of who I truly was, a creation that would begin with a vision of my soul, rather than the random laying down of threads.

I had never given much thought to mystical experiences. Had I been asked, I would have sided with the belief that such experiences were the realm of priests, rabbis, saints, shamans, and swamis. I had no idea that there existed a sizable collection of ordinary people all around the world who had mystical experiences, and that there had always been, and more were having such experiences every day. Nor had I any idea what sort of soil created the fertile ground for this kind of expression of a soul, or that my life was rapidly composting into just the right balance of nutrients for such a development.

Most importantly, I had no idea how difficult it is for our society to accept and understand the nature of such experiences, let alone to offer support and guidance to those of us who stumble into these extraordinary states of mind.

I had a lot to learn.

It was time for this ghostwoman to re-grow her flesh and bones, remember that she mattered, become who she'd always been.

It was time to give up the ghost.

At the hospital I was moved to another stretcher. Once again the bone edges shifted, shooting those fierce daggers through my shin. A shower of glass fell from my clothes onto the crisp white sheet. Emergency room scissors came out and gnawed through my favorite jeans. They fell away from me leaving only a thin hospital gown between me and my bed of broken glass.

Then came my history.

The paramedics had been the first to ask, but they paid it no attention. Now it was the nurse. Soon it would be the resident and the ER physician. Later would come the orthopedist, then the anesthesiologist. "Any medications?"

Chapter 1: Path Finder

I felt those words as if they were a wall, crashing down on me. I was about to lose control of my tears, so the ghostwoman came and rescued me. "I had an injection of eighty-two milligrams of methotrexate yesterday," I answered professionally. This was a drug that stopped the further growth of the embryo I was carrying.

So much for my quiet, personal abortion.

I had to tell everybody about the medicine. It was a toxic drug and I was already frantic about the potential damage my liver had incurred the day before. It would take time to heal. The last thing I needed was another drug to add to its burden, I had to let them know.

To most, my revelation seemed to be just another piece of medical information. My nurse, however, could see past my stoic answers. She read my glistening eyes. As she stood beside me and took my pulse and blood pressure, she looked at me gently and said, "We make the best decisions that we can." And with that, tentatively at first, my tears began to fill the spaces under my eyelids, trickle out the corners, and then converge like a river into a steady flow. My body began a small ruffle of sobbing. I couldn't hold it back.

I shivered under my thin gown and the nurse draped a second blanket over me. How would they get all the bits of glass out of it? I wondered. How do you clean such a thing?

Then the door again opened up, and there were the faces of my family. They looked so worried as they moved into the little room. A smile was the least I could give them. The kids moved closer while Frank stood back behind them, allowing them to be near me. He gave me a little smile of his own. I could see it in the softness of his eyes, and the broadening of his cheeks, though his lips stayed half hidden behind his thick mustache. He was still tanned from our vacation and his newly sprouting, light brown beard complimented his strong jaw and cheek bones. His soft, gray-blue eyes were framed by his glasses and short, straight, sandy colored hair. Old painting clothes emphasized his broad shoulders and lean body. He looked beautiful to me. They all did, they all are.

Iyra had just turned eleven. I couldn't look at her without thinking of how happy and helpful she could have been to a newborn baby brother or sister. And I remembered Jade's comment two years before when I told him he was too big for our baby swing and that we needed to get a bigger one. "No we don't, mommy. You just need to have another baby to put in it!"

Iyra hovered between Frank and me. Her sweet features tightened with fear as she asked how I felt, then told how scared she was to get dropped off at home and have the house wide open and nobody there.

"Can I see your leg?" asked Jade with nine year old fascination. Seeing me sitting up and smiling seemed to wipe any haunting concerns from his face. His big green eyes opened wide, and his lips smiled curiously as he shifted his gaze from my eyes to where my leg was covered by the blanket.

"Sure, but there's not much to see. It's in a splint."

He peeked under the blanket anyway.

"The X-ray's hanging up, though. You can see where it's broken."

Jade looked at the X-ray and his skinny body cringed, shoulders raising, head shrinking back between them. It was easy to see both bones broken severely. "Does it hurt?" he winced.

"Not too bad. I've got ice on it and that keeps it numb. I always thought a broken bone would hurt a lot more than this. But as long as they keep the ice on and don't move me, it hardly hurts at all. How are you? How was school?"

Frank noticed dried blood that covered a gash on my left finger and moved over to that side of the stretcher. He lifted my hand, taking off his glasses so he could examine my wounded knuckle more closely.

Chapter 1: Path Finder

Surprisingly, the little gash was the only cut I received from the accident. Back in the bakery, I thought there'd be far more wounds to contend with, but the apparent bloody mess was just marionberry goo strewn about.

"Looks like it'll need a couple of stitches," he said to me as he continued examining my finger.

Frank is a dentist. To him, a couple stitches has less emotional impact than putting a band aid on a scrape has for me. He offered to sew it up, but I asked him to wait and let the ER doctor take care of it. I wanted him to hold my hand; to tend to my heart, not just my flesh.

Jade's unkempt mass of thick dark curls bounced around the room as he examined all the equipment lying on the counter and hanging on the walls. He chattered nonstop about imaginative ways he could use everything he put his hands on. He opened the drawer at the end of the exam table and picked up a speculum.

"Jade! Mom already told you to stop looking in all the drawers!" Iyra yelled at him. "Those things are supposed to stay clean! Didn't you hear what mom said?"

I had surgery that night, and awoke hours later in the darkness of the early morning. My right knee felt like it was being gnawed through by rats. The morphine drip that hung from a pole to my left might as well have been water, as my pain did not respond to my trembling attempts to increase its flow. I frantically pushed the button calling for the nurse.

"It's not working. I keep trying to turn it up, but it doesn't feel any different."

"It's set for the maximum the doctor ordered."

I paused, remembering my own nights as an intern and the extra fatigue that night calls kept me mired in. But my agony was too great for such thoughtfulness. "Then would you call the resident, please? The pain is unbearable."

I had reached some limit of my pain threshold where my attention was more on myself than my empathy for another. This was a pattern I would begin to repeat, one which forced me to begin growing back into my *self*, ultimately to discover the value and purpose of a healthy ego in the unity of all things.

Frank had called my parents that evening and they'd caught the next flight out to be with me. They were there with Frank and the kids that morning, as I awoke from my half-stuporous, morphine sleep. I was in excruciating pain that first day, and hardly able to carry on a pleasant conversation for more than fifteen minutes.

"Here's your journal," said Frank, handing me the paperback book I'd asked him to bring me. A close friend had given it to me when I began a four-month sabbatical at the beginning of the year. I loved the journal as much for the quotes that were in it as I did for the opportunity to fill the empty spaces with my own thoughts. I'd be in too much pain to write more than half a line later that day. The quote on the page brought me some hope.

Times of growth are beset with difficulties.
They resemble a first birth. But these difficulties arise from
the very profusion of all that is struggling to attain form.
Everything is in motion: therefore if one perseveres
there is a prospect of great success
—I Ching—

Chapter 2
Descent

Frank was working, so Mom and Dad drove me home from the hospital two days later where the 'For Sale' sign stood like an evil sentinel in front of our house. It sucked out my energy just being there and filled me with a deep sadness. We loved our old house, but we'd been looking for another place for two years, since our neighbor began planning to build an apartment complex next door. It was too painful to imagine the old trees being cut down, trading privacy and a park-like feeling for a three story building looming over us ten feet away. But I had changed my mind and I didn't want to move.

Maneuvering myself out of the van, I hobbled with my crutches over the gravel, under the plum trees we had planted almost a decade ago, and through our old wooden gate. The short concrete walkway led to three steps up onto the deep, covered porch. These steps were a little steeper than the practice steps at the hospital, but not a problem. I left the sign behind me for the moment, and crutched into my house.

The sofa was gone. Frank had moved it to the new

Ghostwoman

house, as we'd discussed, while I'd been at the hospital. It left a gaping living room where a hospital bed was to be delivered. It was a hollow room, like the ghostwoman. I could almost feel what was left of my insides drop down and through my feet. Whatever part of my heart had begun to feel comfortable again, due to the surprise visit of my parents, was gone. And I was left as empty as the space I'd just entered.

The hospital bed turned out to be an uncomfortable bother, so after two days of aching back and hips, I sent it all back and returned to our futon upstairs and the warmth of Frank. Throughout the difficulties in our marriage, this part of our relationship was where we could often connect and feel loved. Wrapped in Frank's strength, my tired body felt protected from the world. And I was so chilled, while Frank was like a furnace. He didn't mind me burrowing into his side to get warm, he enjoyed my coolness. In those moments, the balancing influences of our physical bodies would temporarily bridge the sometimes unbearable gap between us emotionally.

We had sort of rushed into the marriage after two years of dating. Frank was my first long-term relationship, and he'd made me feel loved with his persistent desire to be with me. I had been lonely for years, wanted children since the age of about six, and suffered from endometriosis, a disease that carried with it not only excruciating pain, but also the promise of decreased fertility with every passing year. To alleviate the symptoms, I'd had surgery, then taken medication for half a year with side effects of painful muscle cramps, increased hair on my face, arms, and body, and reshaping muscle into more of a man's shape. But within only a couple months of stopping the medicine, the pain returned. Pregnancy was considered another treatment for the condition.

And I loved Frank, I just was not in love with him. I

Chapter 2: Descent

loved him most when we were out in nature where he is most peaceful and himself, but that was only a small part of our life together. Too often, our conversations felt flat and empty. On the day of our wedding, I broke down in tears, confiding to my husband-to-be that I didn't think we had enough in common. He wrapped his arms around my sobbing body and said he would do everything he could to make me happy. I chose to believe his words and intentions. I married the earth with the hope that it would give life to a garden.

    Frank filled the living room void with our old futon. That was where Mom and Dad slept at night, and where I propped myself up for most of my day. From there I could take care of all the household business— the paperwork, the bills, the family schedule. I had volunteer responsibilities for our various schools, and most imminently, there was a letter to write and send off to all eighteen families of Jade's Shabbat school class for a skating event I said I'd help plan.
    I designed a flyer for the empty box that hung below our "For Sale" sign. Dad drove me to get them printed up. I put an ad in the paper for our first open house, which took place the weekend after I returned home.
    And I cried.
    Between the tasks I accomplished, and sometimes during them, I let go rivers of tears. Food tasted like wood. I hugged my children but could not feel them. Another flood would descend.
    I just wanted the earth to swallow me up, to crawl into a hole and never come out. But a parade of visitors began.
    Betsy, my boss, was one of the first to arrive. Mom opened the door while I greeted her from the futon only a few feet away. She was dressed casually. Her gray hair made her look older than the youthfulness of her delicate features. She was an attractive, petite woman in her

forties, with a warm smile and pale blue eyes. Her voice had a soft hum that I'd always found quite pleasant.

She brought some books to share and sat on a dining room chair next to me. She scrunched her face sort of sideways as she asked about my leg, and I told her the details of the accident.

"I don't know if you heard," she answered, "But Lynn broke her leg in the same place only six weeks ago. Both bones, just like you. She was hiking and had to hike out about a half mile with the help of her friends. She's still off work."

It was an odd coincidence to me that I'd never before encountered a patient with a distal tib-fib fracture, and now there were two of us county medical providers with this condition. Stranger still, when I returned to work two months later, I discovered one of my patients had done the same thing to her leg, just by twisting her ankle while she was walking. And another patient told me of her sister, who was hit by a car while she was walking on a sidewalk the same day as my accident. The car just lost control and veered off the road. Her sister was brain dead.

Betsy and I moved on to talking about my house situation, as if breaking a leg wasn't bad enough. "Your colleagues want to get a work party together to help you move," she told me.

"We're not quite ready for that, but thanks for thinking of us," I said. "We have to finish getting this one ready to sell before we can begin to think about the other one. It'll be a little while."

"Just let me know," she answered. Then she asked about the new house. We both had old houses from around the 1920s, and we'd talked many times about enjoying the older styles. "What sort of house is it?"

"It's a 1938 house that was remodeled in the 1970s. It's a contemporary-looking thing, very square with a flat roof. Not the perfect house, but I think it'll be okay. It's in a great setting. Needs a lot of work, but it has potential."

Chapter 2: Descent

I didn't tell her about all the foreboding and panic I had about the house. How I'd wanted to call the whole thing off, but couldn't convince Frank that the house was a big mistake. It was too humiliating, I'd just done that with another house only days before. Dragged him over to see it, talked him into it, then dragged him back to talk him out of it. I'd found the house we bought driving back from revoking our earnest money on another house. I couldn't admit to Frank that I was so stupid to do it twice in a row, though I did try.

After my initial wave of excitement, I could see how much time, money, and energy it would take to turn the weedy grounds into gardens, the cold dark corners into a space where light would flow. I had just started to become interested in holistic medicine and was already unable to find enough time to pursue these studies. "The house costs too much," I said. The endless stream of financial requests from organizations working to solve social and environmental problems stuffed our mailbox daily. It didn't feel right to be spending so much time and money on a house. "I don't think I'll have the time to take care of such a big garden."

I spoke about these things, but I did not stand up for them. I'd changed my mind one too many times to be able to trust it, let alone make a big stink about it. I'd chosen the house for Frank, and in the end, let him make the decision for us. I just signed the papers with trembling hands, feeling like I would vibrate into a million little pieces; page, after page, after page.

Betsy, just mentioning the house, resurrected these memories in a flood. It was a memory of the feeling, more than the events; the feeling of knowing you're making a monstrous mistake, but not being able to do anything about it. Like those awful nightmares where you need to scream, but nothing comes out of your mouth. But I didn't share any of this with Betsy. We weren't that sort of friends.

Ghostwoman

Another day Libbit stopped by and brought us meals for the freezer. Michelle came by with a lasagna. Next, Sandy dropped in. We'd been working in the same office for almost a decade, yet she'd never seen me cry before. Like everyone else, she thought I was crying about the car accident. It was such a blessing to hide behind that trauma.

Lynn came by with her broken leg. Mom got a picture of us sitting on the sofa with our twin casts raised high in the air and smiles on our faces. But it was a few days before the news trickled down to my closest friends.

Cindy came by with hugs and books, then Paula sat with me. And I couldn't hold back, I told her about the abortion. She was the first one besides the staff at the hospital. My tears finally exploded and she moved from the chair and knelt beside me. She wrapped her arms around me and cradled my head close to her. She held me like that for some time, while I cried and cried.

The following day Gorretti brought a stack of moving boxes from her business. A different Cindy from Shabbat School made an eggplant lasagna that I could actually taste. Jade thought it was the best lasagna he'd ever eaten. My rabbi came by. I talked about the house, and how conflicted I felt about spending so much money on a place to live. He reassured me that many people felt this way.

Another mother from Jade's Shabbat School class came one afternoon. She brought us a huge container of homemade soup. She also brought an infant, her seventh child, a beautiful, unplanned blessing.

In Judaism we name our children after someone we love who has died. Some believe this tradition allows the memory to live on. For others, including myself, it is so their spirit could have a body to be reborn into, and a loving family to be a part of. I'd realized that my last period was late the day after we'd learned Frank's gentle grandfather had just had a massive stroke. He died five days later, on Iyra's birthday, the day we closed on the

Chapter 2: Descent

new house, three days before my appointment with my gynecologist.

My sweet Jewish reflections of how new life weaves together the souls of lives gone by, were torn by my understandings of the other realities of life: thirty thousand children dying every day of starvation, millions living in abject poverty, the earth being polluted and degraded by our ignorance of how to collectively live any other way, global warming, resources being devastated and hundreds of creations of God rapidly becoming extinct under the burden of human population. I thought about these things, and balanced them against my limited energy and situation. I had struggled with fatigue *before* I had children, and felt as if I had barely survived raising two of them. How could I handle another one let alone help the mounting situations of our time that threatened the survival of all of us? Frank said he couldn't see himself as the father of a newborn at this point of our life, and I wasn't sure that Frank and I were going to make it in our marriage. I certainly couldn't handle raising another child alone.

I found myself almost wincing at my intelligent friend, thinking she should know better, should understand the consequences of unlimited human population growth. Then I caught myself. Who was I to know what was in the best interest of the world? I had my logical way of thinking, my scientific observations, and the consequences that seemed only too obvious to me. But this was *my* understanding, and this woman was a kind friend of mine and the baby was already here. Who was I to judge that the way she saw her part in the Divine plan was any less correct than my own? She was a wonderful mother.

For me, to have had so many children would have meant I'd given up my hope of humanity finding a balanced place on earth where we, and all of the other creatures could survive. To not have had any children would have been the same sort of testament to a loss of hope. But there is a blurry line between responsibility and faith, and it seems to be different for each of us, sometimes different on different days.

I remembered the words of my nurse, "We make the best decisions that we can."

Then I oohed and ahhed over the beautiful new child, while my friend comforted me about my leg. And we talked about what it takes to make a good pot of soup.

10-9

Sometimes we stumble.

Sometimes we stumble and fall.

And lose our bearings and our wallets, and our self-respect and integrity. But we are still granted life. A life to use as best as we can. To learn with. To care for and revere life. Life, I chose to squash for the good of the whole. A "right" decision? Who will know? But it is a hard one and I am unable to forgive myself for becoming pregnant in the first place.

It is every woman's choice, and should be. But for me, life is so precious. All life.

It's just so sad.

My remorse would not let go, as critical thoughts about all my decisions cycled round and round and round. I broke this cycle briefly one day, as I compared my choices to events in my world that felt senseless and ruthless, but had nothing to do with me.

What about the freak bicycle accident that killed my vivacious, compassionate sister-in-law, so devoted to the service of others? And my dear friend Ruza? Only fifty-five years old, so conscientious about her health, and such

Chapter 2: Descent

a dedicated and excellent physician. She, who had saved countless lives and only wanted to keep doing more, now lay at home dying of cancer. Then there was Leah, a young and healthy pediatrician who suddenly developed a life-threatening infection during her second pregnancy and was forced to abort her much wanted seven month old fetus in order to save her own life.

Was I so much less perfect than God?

* * * * *

Dad helped Frank pack and do odd jobs around the house. He stayed for over a week, long enough to feel stiff from the cool, damp weather. Then he flew home to take care of his own business. It was the first time he and Mom had been apart for more than a night or two since they'd been married. He called her frequently, said he was sleeping with her quilting books to keep him company.

Mom stayed around for over a month. She was my friend, my cook, my housekeeper, my chauffeur, my children's chauffeur, and a wonderful grandmother. Still, for all of our closeness and all my tears I could not bring myself to tell her about the abortion. She drove me to my follow-up gynecology appointments, but I didn't share what they were about. She respected my privacy, too, and didn't ask. Our relationship was the silver lining of those days, as I grew closer to her than I had ever felt before.

Mom nudged me to contact home assistance agencies, refusing to return home to my father until I had a system of help set up. What a chore, all those calls. And the open houses every Sunday. And Frank hurrying through the living room with one box after another.

When he wasn't at work, Frank was fixing up the old house. He pressure washed the outside and the decks, painted the house inside and out, repaired the chimney, restored the porch columns, refinished the door, repaired the gate, and made the landscape immaculate. Once finished, he began moving some of his favorite plants from our overly lush yard to the new place. Trees and rhododendrons he'd lovingly planted over the years, forty to fifty in all. They wouldn't be missed. At the same time, fired with great enthusiasm for the move, he began getting the new place ready.

At meals he'd tell us all his latest accomplishments and what he planned to do next. But he did not talk to me about my sadness, ask how I was feeling, or offer any emotional support. It was as if my despair was an abyss into which he would plummet if he came near. And he was so excited about the new house and had a mountain of work to climb before moving us into the new place.

One evening he brought up an armload of empty boxes from the basement. Four of them went up to the children's room for them to pack up their shelves. He dropped them off, then came back down and began packing up everything that we didn't absolutely need from the living room area, leaving behind a few artistic things for their aesthetic contribution. "Houses sell better when they look less cluttered. It makes them look bigger," he said, turning his full attention on the bookshelves.

I watched the dismantling of my home from the old futon, trying not to feel the pain of my home being dissected. I felt I should be doing more to help, but my legs still swelled a good deal if I didn't keep them up. The bruises were fading but the hard chord in my left leg from a vein that had thrombosed felt like iron, and both swollen knees still felt as though they'd been kicked by a horse.

Frank loped back upstairs, two by two. "You guys haven't packed anything yet! Come on! Get these boxes packed up already!"

Jade pack up his books by himself? He couldn't even put them back on his shelves without rereading every one that touched his hands.

I grabbed my crutches and headed up the stairs.

Chapter 2: Descent

"Need some help?" I asked, peering in from the doorway.

"I don't want to move! I hate that house!" Jade yelled, tears streaming down his beautiful cheeks. I had never seen him so sad before, he was always an expression of exuberance.

"I wish I could just die!" he cried. Then he flopped down on his little futon and buried his head in his blankets.

I had crutched over to the bed by then. Sitting on it with my legs up, I tried to put my arm around Jade but he'd have nothing to do with me. His tears flowed and his little shoulders convulsed with sobs. "You know, Jade," I began quietly. "The new house may not be as wonderful as this one, but it's up off the street and has a big yard. We'll be able to get that dog you two have been wanting. Once we're moved in, we can get a book about dogs and think about what kind we'd like to get. What do you think? Should we get a dog from the pound, or a particular kind of dog?"

At last the sobs began to subside.

"Come on, I'll help you pack up your books." I lifted my cast over to the other side of the low bed, and slid down to the floor. Propped up against the side of the bed, I began to take the books from the case to my right, and neatly put them in the boxes.

10-21-97

I wear my skin inside-out these days. A difficult way to go about life, for one so private as I.

Tears popping out all the time.

I find myself aware of those others out there, who, too, wear their tears in public.

Ghostwoman

> We are a translucent club. We find each other and know...

> A prayer from my little Buddhist book, "Here I am, God. Do what you want with me."
> Perhaps this is my opportunity to understand the Buddhist truth of how attachment causes suffering. Why am I suddenly so attached to the place I've been wanting to move from for the past two years?

While the kids were at school, Frank and I drove to the new house. I was to begin unpacking the boxes Frank had been hauling over and depositing in the various rooms. He was planning to paint. The big flat railing in front of the house was peeling and Frank had decided to take care of it. I found the thought of painting an outdoor railing in November, in Portland, to be a humorous one, but held my tongue. Let him do as he pleases, I thought. He'd painted the old house and enough apartments over the years to know what he was doing.

I crutched inside and up the carpeted entryway stairs that had made me feel like a queen the first time I stepped into the house. I hobbled through the living room, past windows that once held an expansive view, but whose view had somehow caved in and shrunk in my current state of mind. Around the corner and into the small kitchen I paused, staring at the dark, old, commercial flooring with dirt waxed into it; the plain, flat, wooden cabinets that needed refinishing, and the drawers that got stuck if the old dishwasher was open. The oven was so old the handle was Duct-taped together. Dingy gray Formica. You could even see all the dents in the wall where the sheet rock was nailed to the studs.

I crutched my way back around the corner, down the

Chapter 2: Descent

short dark hallway by the tiny bathroom and up the narrow stairway. So many potential places for windows, why did they make it so dark? Why was I seeing so much darkness when at first I saw so much light?

I took the tape measure and began to plan the children's small rooms. I had to carefully lean on one crutch while measuring, as I was still not to put much weight on my broken leg. The other crutch would tumble to the floor periodically, and there was no furniture here yet for me to rest on. Pleasantly, at least, I was surprised to find that the rooms might just work out. We wouldn't need to buy loft beds after all, to fit their furniture underneath. I noticed that Iyra's bedroom door couldn't open fully unless her closet doors were closed.

Who designed this place?

And our room: Frank had boxes of clothes ready for me to unpack in our walk-in closet with the one dim light. I hung some clothes, beginning to get accustomed to leaning on my crutches while hanging things on hangers. I missed the windows in our narrow, old closets.

I had to get out of the darkness. I crutched down the stairs and into the office, which had large windows on two of the sides. There, filled once again with remorse, I couldn't unpack either. Another small room. The half wall of book shelves was completely inadequate for our books, and there was no room for our freestanding shelves. There wasn't a chair in the room, and I quickly became tired of standing on one leg, propped up against the desktop as I unpacked the books. My chest became heavier and heavier.

I crutched out the front door to where Frank was painting.

"I don't like the house," I said, watching his attention focused on his long brush strokes. "I don't think I ever will. I'm sorry I've dragged you and the kids to this place and through all my uncertainty and grief."

Then I sat on the cobbley cement steps and cried.

He paused from his painting for a second and looked up at me. "I think you will," he declared. Then he returned to the white primer and continued to focus on the railing.

I sobbed for some time, though it felt awful to cry in front of Frank, the way he looked through my pain as if it weren't there. Then I stood up on my one "good" leg, picked up my crutches, maneuvered back inside and unpacked.

I found places for the books.

Then I returned home and packed four more boxes.

Accomplishing something felt good, despite how meaningless the whole move felt to me.

> *Look at this window*
> *it is nothing but a hole in the wall,*
> *but because of it, the whole room is full of light.*
> *Being full of light it becomes an influence*
> *by which others are secretly transformed.*
> **—Chuang Tsu—**

Chapter 3
Healing Begins

My mother had left by the time my name surfaced to the top of the therapist's waiting list. Still not driving, I had to ask an acquaintance to drive me to the appointment. I had to ask people for help with all my driving, and it made me squirm. I didn't mind giving help, but hated asking for it.

I had only been to a therapist twice before: two visits to a marriage counselor that spring, where Frank had refused to join me. Before that, I'd tried talking to Frank about what I needed from our relationship. I'd ask him for little things, like paying some attention to me besides in bed, asking me out once in a while, asking me how I was feeling and how I felt about things. He'd tell me he already did this and sometimes a little would change. Then, whatever small changes had taken place would go back to the way they'd been before.

When I noticed our conversations had become confrontational, I began to feel anxious just at just the thought of talking to Frank. I figured at the least we had communication problems we could work on. Frank said he

Ghostwoman

didn't have any communication problems, but if I did, I was free to go by myself. It took me two visits before I could see the lunacy of going to a marriage counselor alone. Now I was seeing someone just for me.

The door to the waiting room opened, and a tall, gray-suited man with matching gray hair, a clean-shaven face, and gentle eyes stood with a pleasant smile. He introduced himself in a warm deep voice.

"Would you like some tea?" he asked as he led me into his office.

"I'd love a cup, thank you," I answered, my eyes beginning to water.

I was the one who offered things to my family. How good it felt for such a little act of kindness to be offered to me. I settled into the leather chair next to the therapist's desk, nervously waiting for him to return.

Dr. Bice had been recommended by a friend. It had taken a month to get in to see him, a long month, during which time I'd regularly looked at antidepressant samples, but never resorted to taking them. Somewhere inside myself I felt like my depression was about something I needed to realize and pull out by its roots. Or perhaps it was something that I needed to bring into my life? I didn't know. I only knew I didn't want some chemical to make me feel happier. I was afraid it might diminish the inspiration I had for uncovering whatever it was that I needed to change. I was still functioning. I didn't need drugs just yet.

Returning to the room, Dr. Bice handed me the tea, then settled into his desk chair. "So what brings you here?" he asked. And it was so awkward to be asked the question I had asked my own patients for so many years. So unnerving, yet at the same time, curiously easy to open up to a total stranger. I rattled off the events of the past two months as succinctly as possible. "I don't know who I am anymore. I don't know what I like, what I want, or

Chapter 3: Healing Begins

what my life is all about. Nothing brings me joy."

"What do you do for yourself?" Dr. Bice asked.

"I like doing things for other people, to help them and make them happy."

"But what do you do to make yourself happy?"

"I've done a little painting once a week, I've enjoyed that over the years. But mostly I do things for other people— my children, my husband, my children's schools. Shouldn't that make me happy?"

He laughed sincerely but without a trace of mockery.

I broke down in tears and couldn't stop for quite some time.

It wasn't that I didn't enjoy doing things for others. It was only that I was empty and tired. I had lived with low energy since my freshman year of college, when I'd come down with a heavy case of mononucleosis. I spent that week sleeping twenty hours a day, and the four hours I was awake were exhausting.

Chewing food felt like lifting weights. I never fully recovered, and subsequently found myself struggling to stay awake in classes, often not succeeding. The summer after college I fell asleep at the wheel of a car. By medical school I couldn't keep my eyes open for more than five minutes in the dark lecture hall. I was nicknamed sperm-head for the way my head would bob and whip back and forth in my sleep as I sat in class, sometimes flinging my pen away with a myoclonic jerk.

Then I'd go home after sleeping all day, take a nap for an hour, awaken to my alarm clock on the other side of the room, have a strong cup of coffee, then go for a swim in a cold pool to wake up. I got my lectures out of class notes and somehow managed to pass all my exams and even do well, to my ongoing great surprise. It felt like God wanted me to become a doctor and was somehow getting me through the process. I just kept putting one foot in front of the other and plodding on.

Ghostwoman

What did I ever do just for the sheer joy of it? What have I ever loved to do that made me feel ALIVE! It took me almost twenty years to discover a passion— DANCING! and it took only four years for my knees to crumble.

God, how I loved to dance. It's just not the same when I can't explode into the music. Staying careful and bent and small is not dancing.

Then there's the fatigue. It's so hard to get into anything when you're tired all the time.

What do I think?

I think I'm too old to be wondering who I am...

...Depressed about the house. Yuck. Until the kids said, "Mom, I love the new house!"

"What do you like about it," I asked.

"Everything!!!!!" And I felt a bit happy, and told them that if they loved the house, then I would grow to love it, too.

11-20-97

Here I am at my 'it will never be a cozy house.'

It is a cold house— its style. Between the fireplace and the sofa is a walkway. It states "look at me but do not get close enough to feel. I am distant and aloof."

It's kind of like Frank and me.

Why doesn't the phone repairman come? He said he'd be here hours ago.

I sit here, my boom box playing music next to me, watching the clouds blowing by. Will this ever feel like home? Home must become a place inside of me.

Chapter 3: Healing Begins

This is not a good day. My birthday. I spent four hours for nothing!

Had to come home to call the phone company, waited over ten minutes to talk to a supervisor. Then I fell apart and sobbed. I feel like I've wasted my time and my life and continue to waste it.

11-21

My birthday evolved much better than it began. I figured out the problem with the phone (contacts), then Frank finished working early and we all shared a great meal at Marrakash. After celebrating so many years in that restaurant, it feels like a second home. The food, the service with the same waiter, the atmosphere, all so inviting and so exotic it is at the same time, homey and transcendent!

Frank lost his temper with the kids, but we (the kids and I) worked through that at bedtime. None of us are perfect.

I awoke around 3 am. Came downstairs for a cup of tea and some leftover crisp. Such a lovely and quiet time of the day in this old house. No traffic noises yet, only the sweet songs of the birds awakening.

While lying in bed I thought about how Frank talks to me that feels so unpleasant. He addresses my depression and confusion by telling me what to do and think. This only alienates me from whatever he's saying.

I hope someday I can help him understand what feels good— to just ask, then listen with empathy.

Ghostwoman

Offer any opinions as h<u>is</u> opinion, not as if his opinions are the ultimate wisdom that I need to follow.

> To understand truth
> one must have a very sharp, precise, clear mind;
> not a cunning mind, but a mind capable of looking
> without any distortion, a mind innocent and vulnerable.
> Only such a mind can see what truth is.
> —J. Krishnamurti—

Over the next few weeks, Dr. Bice gently listened to my despair. When I tried to bury it before I understood it, he drew it out. He helped me see all my emotions as being worthy. He did not reject me for my tears. Though the feelings themselves felt awful, and revealing them felt embarrassing, having them validated felt strangely good. Not good enough to stay in these more gloomy states of mind, but good enough to work through them with a gentleness toward myself.

I also talked about the meaning of life, and health, and my work and frustrations about work. I was tired of treating people's symptoms and tired of having so little to offer the many who suffered so much.

"Have you ever heard of Caroline Myss?" Dr. Bice asked.

"Who?"

"Caroline Myss. It's pronounced 'mace,' but spelled M-y-s-s. She's written a couple of books about the universal spiritual causes for physical and mental illness. She'll be in Seattle giving a workshop in January."

He showed me a brochure. The workshop was a seminar about her book, *Anatomy of the Spirit*. I thanked him for the information, but knew that I was not in the market to be conferencing in Seattle or anywhere else,

Chapter 3: Healing Begins

with our double mortgage. But I was intrigued enough to stop at the library on my way home and put my name on a waiting list for the book.

Two weeks later I was reading passionately. First it was *Anatomy of the Spirit*. Next came *The Wisdom of Healing*, by David Simon, M.D., about Ayurvedic medicine, the ancient East Indian holistic medical tradition. Simultaneously I read a book on Jewish mysticism, *Stalking Elijah*, by Roger Kamenetz. I resonated with the sixteenth chapter, 'The Door of Pain,' which seemed to be a necessary entryway to some vital understanding that could not be accessed in any other way.

With my books in hand, waiting in my various doctor's offices no longer irritated me, but became cherished time, the longer the better. Otherwise my reading was sandwiched in between conferences with teachers, with the middle-school principal to consider where Iyra would go to school next year, with the neighborhood elementary-school principal as I began planning where to put Jade after his three years of Montessori were over, and with training a new home aide after the last one made off with my favorite hat and never showed up again.

By that time I was reading about the importance of forgiveness and letting go, for the process of healing. Not quite understanding the whole picture, I blew off any follow-up on the little hat indiscretion.

Jade began his drum lessons. Iyra continued her music lessons across town. Always, there were the groceries to be bought, and meals to be prepared. With Frank's suggestion and lack of time to be my chauffeur, I was driving with my left foot by then.

The phone broke again and it took a week before the phone company could fix the problem for good. Then there was Jade's birthday that needed to be planned. Thanksgiving. Chanukah for my family, and Christmas for Frank's.

Ghostwoman

I decided to return to the discount bookstore to buy a couple copies of the treasures I'd discovered, to give as presents. There were no more copies of the ones I was looking for, but another caught my eye, *The Path to Love*, by Deepak Chopra MD, *A Guide to Spiritual Self-Healing*. I picked it up for myself.

Appointment with my orthopedist: the bones weren't showing signs of healing yet.

With my gynecologist: doing fine.

A series of appointments with an acupuncturist I had just started seeing: her herbs and needles were doing something; my bones didn't stick out so far and I'd been less depressed.

With a homeopath recommended by my pharmacist: he helped me begin to find peace with my abortion, and begin to let go of my unnecessary negative judgment about it. Then he gave me a constitutional remedy for everything.

Frank scrubbed the kitchen in the new house, futilely trying to get the waxed-in rings of dirt off the floor. He oiled the flat cabinets out of their dingy finish until they glowed and smelled of orange peel.

I talked with my auto insurance company, which was dealing with the insurance company of the woman who'd hit me. This seemed ridiculous since I wasn't in my car during my accident, but it was the way they handled these things. And I began, because of my father's strong recommendation, to work with a lawyer on the accident issues.

I was tired.

Another appointment with the orthopedist. Still no sign of healing on the X-ray and it had been almost two months since the accident. "You need to stress it more," he told me. "It's time to walk on it to stimulate the bones to grow. Just use one crutch now."

"Does that mean I can go back to work?" I asked.

"That would be fine. The more you can be on it, the

Chapter 3: Healing Begins

better it'll heal. Just be sure to put it up if it swells."

Stopping by the desk to schedule my next appointment, I discovered none of the bills had been paid. I didn't understand. The husband of the woman who crashed into me, Mr. Bloom, had called and spoken to Frank when I was in the hospital. He said they had plenty of insurance and everything would be taken care of. The Blooms had even sent me flowers.

* * * * *

We moved into the new house on Thanksgiving weekend, the day after Jade's ninth birthday party. Frank did most of the work and his friends helped with the heaviest pieces.

Outside, it was cold, gray, and raining, a perfect mirror for the state of my heart, though I did my best to be thankful and keep a positive attitude in my head.

I made a pot of chicken chili for lunch for us all, the first cooked meal in the "new" kitchen.

One week later I was back at work, and it felt more like home than home did. Marie, my nurse, met me with an exuberant hug. I felt so warm and loved, so appreciated for who I was. Throughout the day the staff and my colleagues dropped by to welcome me back and visit for as long as we were able.

Since I was still on crutches and had been away for awhile, I had a light schedule and was able to spend more time with each patient. I couldn't help but recognize the patterns of psychospiritual causes for illness, as outlined in Dr. Myss' work. I was particularly aware of this in my established patients who I knew quite well, and whose chronic conditions I'd been following for years. Based on my reading, I began a bit of psychospiritual counseling wherever I thought it might be welcomed and helpful. It was very appreciated, and work never felt better. None of my patients who previously had felt so hopeless to me felt

Ghostwoman

hopeless anymore. I had something new to offer that might help. But I was scheduled for only four more half-days before we left for our long-planned Christmas vacation.

Back at home, Frank cleaned the carpets and the old sofa, then began working on landscaping the new place in earnest. I attended to the usual housework, as my allotment for home care was used up, then slowed down to put together Chanukah treats for Jade's class: thirty little dreidles, each with two pieces of chocolate *gelt* (coins), wrapped in colorful Chanukah paper. I'd offered to do a little presentation, the same one I had been doing in my children's classes since they were in kindergarten. I was not about to let a pair of crutches stop me from what was probably my last year. The kids were getting a little old for this.

The children all gathered around me on the floor of the spacious Montessori classroom while I sat on a chair in front of a low wooden table. Jade enjoyed the place of honor, passing out the little presents to his classmates while I prepared the candles. All those precious, chattering, little bodies became mesmerized and silent as I broke the fire marshal's laws by lighting the candles, then started singing the melodious Hebrew blessings over the light.

I explained the meaning of the Hebrew, then pulled out our favorite Chanukah story to read, *The Chanukah Guest*, by Eric Kimmel. But before beginning the funny story, I gave the children a synopsis of the real Chanukah story, the story of the battle the Jewish people fought for religious freedom over two thousand years ago. Then we talked about how America was founded by Europeans who were searching for the same kind of freedom.

I didn't have time to explain the way the latter happened at the eventual expense of the freedom of the people who already lived here, and the parallels to my own Jewish history. We didn't have time to talk about the way history was full of moments to be proud of, as well as

Chapter 3: Healing Begins

experiences to learn from. I just moved right into the funny story about the old grandmother who was almost blind and deaf, and who mistook a wandering bear for the local rabbi. Laughter bubbled from the bobbing children. Even Jade, who'd heard the story at least a dozen times, could hardly stop cackling.

* * * * *

Days later we landed in California, where Eve, Frank's mother, was at the airport terminal waiting for us. None of this, "I'll pick you up at the baggage claim" stuff. She couldn't wait to see the children!

"Grandma!!!" The kids ran into her arms and squeezed her tightly. Eve smiled radiantly and her eyes sparkled joy. She laughed a lyrical, light, soprano laugh. She looked up at Frank and me. "Hi Harriet, hi Frank," she said with a slightly more reserved tone.

We weren't going to come back for a while after last year. It had been a rough visit. They'd been getting progressively worse for the past four years since Frank's sister got run over by the truck. Before then we looked forward to flying down every year for Christmas. My family was back east and celebrated Chanukah, which isn't a major Jewish holiday. But Christmas was Frank's family's celebration and a marvelous time. We loved hanging out with Frank's mom while she happily cooked for us all. His grandparents, mostly Oma, baking panfuls of strudel and kipful. Frank's wonderful brothers and sisters and all those beautiful nieces and nephews we watched grow up together. Amusement parks, the beach, and their favorite— the neighborhood rocket ship park with it's wildly imaginative and expansive playground. It was one grand party full of love, day after day.

Until Susan died. And every year since then was a little bit worse. The last Christmas was unbearable.

I had brought Eve a book on post traumatic stress

Ghostwoman

disorder and that was the end of a ten-year, beautiful relationship. The book spoke of the normality of emotional difficulties after going through what Eve had experienced, but I might as well have given her a vial of poison for the way she reacted. From then on she either ignored me, or flung criticisms and insults my way. I didn't know what to do about it, so I said and did nothing. I knew it was her own pain she was flinging at me, so I just tried to let it roll off my back.

Frank told me it had been like that for him, off and on, the whole time he was growing up. His dad had tried to get Eve to get some help but she refused. She could never acknowledge that she had any problems, as if the stigma of mental, or emotional illness, was so dreadful that she couldn't even consider it.

I had known for some time that Eve was a child during World War II, when her family's farm was taken by the Serbs and the Russians. Her family, ethnic Germans living in Yugoslavia, were either murdered or placed in concentration camps.

She didn't talk about it, but Oma and Opa would share some of the stories. Most were gruesome, but some were stories of how their Serbian friends saved them, or how Opa was forced to fight on both sides of the war, but never killed another human being. I figured the death of Susan tore open Eve's old emotional wounds. But I didn't dare mention it again.

It was ironic to me that my family is the Jewish one, and Frank's is German, yet his is the one with the deep scars from the war. I always knew it didn't matter what you are. It's not about being anything. It's just about fear and hurt and need, and making someone else feel small so you can feel bigger, or making someone feel bad because you do, most often unconsciously.

But there we were, visiting again. Oma was so sad since Opa died, and with my accident and all, we hadn't made it down for the memorial service. I thought maybe

Chapter 3: Healing Begins

with my broken leg, Eve would have some sympathy towards me that would counter her animosity. She had a compassionate and giving heart, which was all I had known of her for the first ten years we knew each other. She was the generous, loving soul, who flew up to take care of me for a month after each of my children was born. She'd unobtrusively cook and clean for us while I was at work, even wake up in the middle of the night to bring the baby to me to nurse so I wouldn't have to get out of bed! And she listened to my troubles with Frank that were going on even back in those days.

Frank and I stayed at Oma's apartment, which was just around the corner from Eve's place. That gave Oma company, and a little more room for us. It also gave me the privacy I needed to begin meditating, my personal goal for the vacation. I could find quiet at Oma's that was impossible when the kids were around. And with Eve taking care of meals for all of us, and treasuring her time alone with the kids, I'd have the time I needed to begin a practice.

All the books I'd been reading talked about how important meditation was for healing. In the Ayurvedic tradition, it holds a place of importance right up there with diet and exercise. Since my bones seemed to be taking their sweet time growing back together again, and I was still an emotional mess (though I could control myself in public by then), I figured it would do me some good.

I wanted to give it a try back at home, but hadn't been able to find the time when everything was so busy. Here, with Eve's help, I could carve out the time I needed. And since the air between us was still pretty thick, I didn't think she'd miss me when I was gone.

The night after we arrived I excused myself from the playful chaos of Eve's apartment after dinner and crutched back to Oma's to give it a try. The little porch light was on, as well as the light in the small entryway. I hobbled through the little kitchen, and pulled a chair into

Ghostwoman

the adjacent dark living room.

Following the instructions in Dr. Simon's book, I sat comfortably erect, rested my hands in my lap, and closed my eyes. From there I followed my breath. It began with the awareness that each inhalation begins in the belly, with the belly relaxing outwards. Soft belly. Just being aware and allowing the breath. I felt the air fill my lungs from the bottom up, slowly filling my chest until it reached the uppermost portions inside and below my shoulders. I shared this awareness with the cool sensations my nostrils felt during the in-breath. Then I followed my breath in reverse, feeling the warm out-breath and some muscles letting go, others tightening. My goal was to think of nothing but my breath, to let go of my thoughts, to notice them if they came up, observe them, give them a name, and with the next exhalation, blow them away and refocus on my breath.

That was all. Just focusing on my complete breaths, and witnessing my thoughts and feelings without judgment or analysis, just blowing them away.

Oma came home about fifteen minutes after I began. I could hear her rattling the heavy screen door, then quietly walking through the kitchen. I could feel her petite body coming my way as it navigated it's familiar territory.

"Hi, Oma," I said quietly, not wanting to startle her, but startling her anyway.

"Oh! You scared me! I didn't know you verr in here. I thought you'd gone to bed!" she said to me in her German-accented voice. "Do you vant me to turn the light on?"

"No thanks. I don't need it. I'm just sitting here with my eyes closed. I'll only be another fifteen minutes."

"Take as much time as you vant. I'll get out of your vay. I'm sorry to disturb you. I didn't know you verr in heerre," she said apologetically.

"That's OK," I smiled to her. "I'm learning how to meditate."

"That's good!" she smiled back. "I'll leave you

Chapter 3: Healing Begins

alone." And she disappeared into the room with the television set, thoughtfully closing the door.

I was committed to my practice for twenty to thirty minutes twice every day, once in the morning, and once every night (though I'd usually fall asleep sitting up at the end of the day). This was what was recommended, and who was I to argue? I knew nothing about meditation except what I had read, and previous books seemed to have been in agreement with both this technique and with the need for diligence in daily practice, ideally twice a day.

Besides, it took only days for me to appreciate meditation just for its own sake. To have a goal of *not* having to figure anything out, not evaluating or judging, was the reprieve I desperately needed. My unpleasant ruminations lost their importance during meditation. My lack of feeling any meaning in my life was asked to wait. It was time just to breathe, and in just breathing I was achieving some rightness in these moments.

Even Oma quieted her chattering and allowed me my quiet time and space. I thought it cute the way she would say to others not to disturb me, that I was praying. I suppose they are sort of the same, but in prayer, I do the talking. In meditation, I let go of any need to speak. I just listen, *Shema*. The Hebrew word that begins the central prayer of my Judaism, *Shema*. Listen Israel, God, Your God, is One.

Meditation also gave me a break from feeling miserable about how things were going with Frank. He was keeping his distance, and I was miserable about it. Though much improved with my depression, I needed someone to care about me and hold me with love, to ask how my leg was holding up after long days at the amusement park. But none of that happened, and with unresolved birth control issues, we no longer even shared closeness in our bed. Meditation embraced me when no

Ghostwoman

one else would.

Back at home, Frank's distance was understandable because he was so busy with the houses and with his work. It seemed quite reasonable that he'd have no time for me, so I didn't expect much. My therapist and my friends kept me afloat, not to mention my books and my journal. But on vacation, all we had was time.

I got up my nerve to talk to Frank one morning. We were getting ready to go over to Eve's for breakfast. We hadn't been talking to each other, just gathering our things in silence. I was talking silently to myself, however, trying to inspire my courage, making our impending conversation up in my head as I was so skilled at doing. Those conversations were all so perfect and flowed so effortlessly. It was too bad they were so seldom expressed. Past failures were the mortar that built the walls to my free expression, though I wanted to tear them down. Taking a deep breath, I told Frank I needed a little attention and affection. I needed some hugs, to feel like he cared about me, not just the house.

He paused to listen, but kept his distance, standing three feet away in Oma's small bedroom. Revealing no emotion, he told me he couldn't touch me without feeling aroused. And since I wouldn't let him come near me without a condom, which he hated, he needed to keep his distance.

I wasn't talking about sex, and his response took me by such surprise that my mind went blank as it always did when I was confronted with something unexpected.

I felt hopeless about Frank and me. But I didn't give up.

I kept meditating.

Shortly after we returned from California, I brought it up again. I had to, nothing would stay buried anymore. The initial feelings of serenity that had accompanied my meditation had metamorphosed. I'd quiet my mind, only

Chapter 3: Healing Begins

to have feelings of profound sadness erupt, as though my heart were retching.

Loneliness. Stark loneliness. The feeling that I was isolated in a separate cocoon from everything and everyone.

I hadn't cried for almost a month, so was a bit surprised by the intensity of my emotions, as my tears flowed like some forgotten faucet. But I was learning not to judge or to block anything. I just observed, refocused on my breathing, and found my mood somewhat lifted by simply stepping back from my emotions into an objective awareness of them.

The clarity of this realization lifted my spirits enough to slow the tears. It was as if I'd been fighting some demon in the dark, and now the lights were on. It gave me something that I could work with, and my hopelessness began to drain away.

I walked downstairs, eyes all puffy and red. Frank was sitting at the kitchen table reading a magazine. I stood in the doorway and I told him about my experience, about the insight that I had just received about how lonely I was.

He looked up and listened, but did not know what to say, so he made no move to comfort me.

Chapter 4
The Next Three Months

Work kept my spirits up. I loved the research connecting psychospiritual reality with physical reality, and I continued to include this counseling with a number of patients I'd been working with for years, and knew quite well. Trudy was one of these early encounters. She was a short, thirty-five-year-old woman, who weighed almost three hundred and fifty pounds. Knee and back trouble along with generalized weakness following a long hospitalization for severe infection, had left her in a wheelchair.

I always enjoyed seeing Trudy. No matter how little I had to offer her for her numerous problems, she always seemed grateful for the time we spent together. She was a remarkably compassionate woman, with a tendency to allow others to treat her poorly without standing up for herself. She'd come from an abusive childhood and was in counseling to try to work through her many issues.

Living with her boyfriend gave her a place to stay in exchange for absorbing his verbal insults and criticisms. It also gave her a place to learn to speak up for herself and

Chapter 4: The Next Three Months

set her limits, but it was a slow process with frequent backsliding.

Prior to my Christmas break, I had seen Trudy for follow-up visits from her latest series of hospitalizations. While I was recuperating with my broken leg, she had been in the intensive care unit for a leg infection. Trudy held large quantities of fluids in her feet and legs and had been plagued by chronic infections and skin ulcers for the preceding two years. Her infections had become resistant to all the standard oral antibiotics, and her last episode had spread into her blood, threatening her life. When I saw Trudy she was two-and-a-half weeks out of the hospital and was being cared for by a visiting nurse who checked on her daily. She was in her last week of a long course of antibiotics.

She greeted me from her wheelchair with a warm smile and eyes that glistened with both joy and pain.

"Dr. Cohen! I'm so glad you're back! I heard about your accident; how horrible! How's your leg?"

"It's doing O.K. Needs me to walk on it to get it to heal, which is good, because I've missed work. Thanks for asking about me. But what about you? I see you've been through quite a bit since I last saw you. How are you feeling? Tell me about *your* legs." I asked.

"They've been starting to burn again like they did last time. But I'm still taking the antibiotics," she reassured me.

I looked at her legs. They looked awful— swollen and fiery red, a clear sign that the cellulitis was back. I didn't want to have to put her back into the hospital for more antibiotics if I could at all avoid it. She needed to save those medications for a last resort if, God forbid, it spread to her blood again. We had to try to keep her from becoming resistant to everything.

"Trudy," I began. "What's going on? Your legs had been doing so well before I left. What's different?"

She thought a few moments before answering.

"I guess I'd been keeping them elevated more," she answered.

"Why can't you keep them elevated now?"

Her gaze dropped to the floor. "Fred tells me I'm lazy if I'm down for more than an hour or two, so I get up and try to do something around the house. He's not too well himself, you know."

I'd been following Trudy and her relationship with Fred for some time. She'd move in, she'd move out. Her self-esteem would flourish for a few days, then melt down. "That's going to kill you," I said softly, knowing I was stating the situation strongly, but knowing also that unless Trudy took care of herself, her infection would worsen and spread as it did before and she could very well die. We didn't have the luxury of time to work with her therapist to help her to stand up for her own needs. Besides, she needed more than that. She needed to feel cared about and loved.

"You need to find a different place to stay. Tonight. Somewhere where you feel allowed to stay off of your feet and keep them elevated until they're well. Is there anywhere you can go? Any friend you can stay with who can help take care of you for a while?"

Trudy assured me she'd keep her legs elevated. I doubted whether that would be enough at this time, but I was at a loss for what to recommend from my conventional therapies. I flashed on some of the Ayurvedic principals I'd just been reading about, and decided to give it a try.

I knew from my years of working with Trudy that she was *kapha*, one of the three major personality/body types that Ayurvedic medicine identifies. I decided to recommend the daily oil massage of her feet and legs with olive oil, which I remembered to be the oil most beneficial for *kapha* types. "Stop the other stuff you're using and let's give this a try. And call me right away if you get any worse."

Chapter 4: The Next Three Months

I left the exam room and limped to the nursing station. I found my nurse and asked her to call in the change of orders for Trudy's visiting nurse.

"Olive oil?" she looked at me curiously.

"What she's using isn't working and I've been reading about the use of olive oil. Thought we'd try it. Oh, and also have the visiting nurse massage the oil into Trudy's feet after she takes care of the leg ulcers."

We were lucky that Trudy had a nurse coming out daily. Between her back and her weight it would have been totally impossible for Trudy to massage the oil into her own feet, one of the recommended practices in Ayurvedic health maintenance.

By the following week, Trudy had moved in with a friend and her legs were starting to improve.

When I saw Trudy for a follow-up appointment two weeks later, even her chronic ulcers were gone! Was it the olive oil? The change in environment from a critical one to a supportive and nurturing one? I believed it was both, and was inspired to continue this new line of counseling and treatment that had been so successful.

Between my meditation, and return to work, my own emotional and physical health settled down. Even my bones started to heal and I was able to switch to a removable air cast. Then it was Frank's moods that began to dominate our life.

He was returning to the patterns I'd been struggling with before our move began. It seemed as if his issues had been put into neutral with his excitement about the house and the monstrous task of moving. Now that we were almost back to plain old life again, Frank's anger was resurfacing. Days would pass where he would look at us with an icy stare, unsmiling, noticing only our shortcomings and imperfections, unable to notice, or at least comment positively about us, or our accomplishments of the day. I tried to talk to him about it briefly. I'd tried to talk to him about it many times over the years.

Ghostwoman

I told him I couldn't survive in a relationship that was so cold.

"I'll try to smile," he said, his face unchanging.

11:15 pm

Shabbat. I sit by the wood stove and warm my back. Tea steeping. I need echinacea. I think I'm getting a cold.

They are all in bed and asleep.

And I was HAPPY today. Periods of great happiness. And dinner was peaceful and sweet. The children were so fun, and no bickering for a change!

I lit the candles. So special in the winter when it's dark outside. We all said the blessing over the light, then raised our glasses and blessed the fruit of the vine. Cut the bread. Said the Chamotzi.

Then, on a lark I decided to do the blessings over the children, which I so rarely remember to do since I wasn't brought up with that ritual, sweet as it is.

I walked over to Iyra and placed my hands on her head. I didn't use the standard blessing, I don't know the words. Besides, I wanted to give her a blessing in my own words. Health and happiness. Courage. Abundance of love, and that all her needs are met and then some. Then I added that she would love sharing her abundance with others.

From there I moved over to Jade, who rarely appreciates affectionate gestures from me. This day he did not try to brush away my hands or scoot away. He closed his eyes for a moment. I could see his face reflected in the glass. It was contorting

Chapter 4: The Next Three Months

into goofy expressions. I blessed him with similar goodies, adding the wish that he be able to invent all those wonderful contraptions he's always inventing in his head some day, and that they be a benefit to the happiness and health of not only himself and his family, but to all the people in the world.

    I moved on to Frank, blessing him with happiness and contentment with his life, few difficult patients, assistants who understood the need for sterile technique and wouldn't get wigged out if he corrected them about it, that his garden would thrive, and he have plenty of time for piano playing and kayaking.

    Then I sat down, and Iyra spoke up with a blessing for us all. Then Jade, too, joined the blessing game. Frank sat silently.

1-10-98

    Where I live is not nearly so important as how I live.

    Still, the morning here was so beautiful. From the bedroom window I watched a sea of fog engulfing the valley below. The fir trees tiptoed out of the sea. And above, a soft purple blue morning was embraced by wafts of pink.

    As I watched, the fog sea rose, and off and on, enveloped us in a blanket of soft blur. Finally it lifted further, revealing the clarity of this beautiful day.

    This was my morning meditation, too lovely for me to close my eyes.

Ghostwoman

Jan. 11

Snowing. The children outside sledding. Frank shoveling the driveway, and it is supposed to do this again tomorrow.

Cancel swim meet. Cancel Frank's kayaking. Cancel my Shabbat School meeting. Enter a day without power, but with the warmth of a wood stove.

An article I'm reading, "Yoga and Meditation and the Ego," helped me to have some hope about my relationship with Frank. My meditation practice, too, no matter how meager, helps. I was asking more of Frank than he could do/be, yet, that day. It seemed so simple to me— so impossible for him. I thought it was choice, but perhaps I was wrong.

Do we get ourselves into more trouble thinking? or not thinking?

Thought needs to be, but always balanced with feeling and sensitivity. For self AND others.

The children sled down the front yard in their plastic toboggans. A gentle slope. Frank shovels ramps and creates jumps for them.

I have fun watching him from the living room window. He's a good father. Together we can be more than either of us alone.

How far I've come from yesterday morning when a part of me thought I should start packing, had no choice, wanting nurturing, emotional intimacy, and sweet, loving, touch so desperately.

1-17-98

A tense day. I awoke depressed. I missed my meditation yesterday. Today I found the time but

Chapter 4: The Next Three Months

lost the way. It's harder now that I'm back to work. No time to bathe my psyche regularly in all those books and words and loving wisdom.

Why am I visited by still more sadness? It's not so bad, this house, this marriage. Why is it so hard for me to lighten up? Frank's been very sweet lately. He smiles at us all and has been a bit more affectionate since I talked to him.

The lawyer calls started coming in about the time the oven broke down. The woman who'd hit me was claiming she had a seizure. Under Oregon law, that meant that she wasn't negligent. The accident became an act of God.

The thought that one could crash into a bakery, break someone's leg, and then take a position that would absolve any responsibility for the accident, was difficult for me to accept. Her husband was a lawyer. I wondered whether she'd caught her disorder from him? Or perhaps it was their insurance company that was calling the shots.

Cynicism battled with my desire to give the Blooms the benefit of the doubt, and my cynicism was winning. Such thoughts were fueled by the yet unresolved detail of the cell phone cord my bakers had found in the wreckage. No one had claimed it, but it had to come from somewhere.

My lawyer had subpoenaed the Blooms for their cell phone records. We'd know soon enough.

My hospital and doctor bills were at least getting paid by my auto insurance.

"It looks like we're going to need to file a lawsuit," my lawyer advised.

A lawsuit? None of my healing books talked about lawsuits. They all talked about forgiveness, and acceptance, and letting go. They also talked about honoring oneself and honesty.

Ghostwoman

1-28

Iyra and Jade are so wonderful. They take turns comforting me when I'm sad. Their hugs. Their words. Today it was Iyra who was so whole, so complete. At eleven, she brushes off criticisms like flies, which of course stick to me like flypaper!

She comforts my tears and says, "go ahead and cry, Mommy, it's O.K."

2-3

Strange happenings.

A beautiful, sunny, winter day. Driving to work I was listening to Caroline Myss' audio tapes. She was telling a true story that included a powerful dream, and it set off powerful sobbing on my part. How convenient that I had my appointment with Dr. Bice today. He asked me about my own dreams. I began with one I remembered from my childhood, when I was around five or so. It was a recurrent dream. The ballerina dancing in space. She was surrounded by darkness, I couldn't tell if there was a ceiling or a floor, there was just this ballerina in a pink tutu, dancing gracefully in blackness. Then as she extended her arm, it came apart from her body. Her legs, one, by one in elegant extension, floated away. Piece by piece she came apart and I awoke in fear, with my heart racing.

I was about fourteen when I had the dream about the torture chamber. Everything was dark and cold and gray. I was a wall in this chamber. I don't remember seeing anything, but I could hear the

Chapter 4: The Next Three Months

screams, and I could feel their vibrations. I woke up petrified and shaking all over.

Then the dream where I was in a house where I often baby-sat, in a suburban south Florida neighborhood. I opened the front door to the house and a large vicious dog was outside and it lunged at my throat.

"Frightening dreams. Do you remember any others?"

I was almost embarrassed to tell him the next dream that popped into my head. I never told anyone this one before and hadn't thought about it since I was a child.

It was a dream I had when I was between seven and ten years old. In it I was writing, writing, writing, everything that would help all the problems in the world— lead the world toward peace. In that one dream I wrote hundreds of pages. It was so real.

I wonder what the dream I've been having lately is all about? I've had a different version of it a number of times. I'm back in another town. Alone. Working in a hospital, but I've forgotten how. And the place is unfamiliar. I'm observing. Or am I? Different dreams, slightly different settings, always trying to help sick people. Always alone. Never knowing what I'm doing. Scary.

It was time for me to coordinate the multicultural fair at Jade's school. I had created and coordinated this event the year before, and thought it would be easier getting it off the ground the second year. The director had been so supportive, and the teachers and parents had given me such positive feedback.

"Flyer? Multicultural fair? What flyer?" I was asked as I followed up the third flyer with telephone calls to all the parents.

"It's a multicultural fair to promote an appreciation of our diverse heritages," I answered. Then the cajoling and nudging. A reminder to one family that they were the only African-American family in the school. "It's so important for you to be there and share your family's roots and experiences."

And to others, "What do you mean you're not multicultural? Every person comes from somewhere and has a story and a heritage. This is a great chance for you and your daughter to explore this together...."

"Nobody is just white. Nobody is just anything. We're all something special."

The previous year I had taught an Israeli folk dance to each of the classrooms, which they performed as part of this event. But this year that option was out of the question. One of the other mothers was going to teach traditional dances from India, and that would be enough. But my leg was feeling a little better, and the children who loved the Israeli folk dancing kept asking me when they would be able to dance with me again. I broke down and agreed to teach my son's class one dance that many of them still remembered, then invited the interested children from the other class to join us. As long as I didn't hop on that foot, and my air cast was cinched tight, my leg could handle it.

Frank was working on the front yard when I came home. I watched him as I drove up the long narrow driveway. He had finished pulling up the ivy from the slope in front of the house and was planting the rest of the trees he'd moved over from the old house. I parked the van, then took the time to walk along the path around the house and notice all the work he'd been doing.

Chapter 4: The Next Three Months

The front slope was looking much less bare now that he had the trees and rhodies in. A small sea of bulbs had sprouted, unexpected buried treasure that I could not wait to see in bloom. Walking around the house on the cement path, I admired his work, finally pausing at the side of the house where he'd pulled out the old dead juniper and had planted the Clareodendron suckers that had sprouted in the middle of the yard at the old house. Here they'd grow fast and shade the southern windows within three years. For now, in their leafless winter garb, they looked like five sticks evenly spaced.

It looked so artificial.

"Looks so much better!" I said to him. "But... they're spaced so evenly it doesn't look very natural. Would you mind moving that one a little over this way, and perhaps putting a rhodie in between those two? It would break it up a little."

"Harriet, I'm not moving the trees or the rhodie. Do you know how much those things weigh? They're staying where I planted them. They'll look fine."

I said no more that day about the garden. The trees *were* heavy, and Frank had put a lot of work into the yard. He was dealing with his carpal tunnel syndrome on top of that, and with my leg still in a cast, I wasn't able to step on a shovel and make any contributions.

But the next time I was out in the yard I noticed that the rhodie and two of the trees had been moved.

3-15-98

Life has been busy, but flowing fairly smoothly. My Shabbat school commitments done, the multicultural fair for Jade's school, done, and everyone is THRILLED with the puppy Frank brought home this week. I don't know how he managed the stick shift with his hand all bandaged up from his surgery

Ghostwoman

just two days before. He still lets me drive the automatic with my wimpy leg. And driving home 30 miles with the little puppy in his lap, he is amazing when he gets his mind set on something. Said he figured he'd have time to train her while he was off work recuperating from the surgery. Wish I felt he loved me as much as he loves the dog. He can't walk by her without bending down to give her a snuggle and a hug. She's awfully cute, though. Her name is Mondeau. She's a golden retriever and such a sweet thing. I can see why the kids and Frank are so in love with her.

Today began smoothly enough. Good book, good talks with friends. Iyra's swim meet, home, meditating on the heart.

Led to a flood of tears. AGAIN!

Feelings of dead ends. Wherever I look --> dead ends. Joy feels stunted. Everything I do, I do to get "it" done. "It" changes, but not the feeling behind it. There is always a long line of things that are waiting to be done next. The laundry piles up. The refrigerator empties out, the mail piles up. No one else even answers the voice mail anymore but me. Someone is always there needing something. The kids or the commitments or the community. Spend time fixing something nice and it's gone. Back to square one.

Same old same old.

My life— work until I die. Get it done. Get it done. There is no time to appreciate anything in this life of mine. Sleep is interrupted by an alarm. Shower is rushed. Breakfast is rushed. I'm late.

Chapter 4: The Next Three Months

Patient after patient. Never enough time for them, they deserve more. Always rushed. No time to eat, no time to pee. Time to pick up the kids. Time to rush off to one of their classes. Time to squeeze in the groceries. Pick up the pile of mail. All these people that want my time and money. All the causes that need more time and money. They pile up on my desk as I go into the kitchen to begin dinner. Put in a load of clothes on the way. Put dinner on hold. Run to pick up one child. Go back to dinner. Run to pick up second child. "Do you have any homework? It's time to practice your drums. You haven't practiced your cello. Would someone else please answer the phone? Almost everything I FEEL is work.

I work harder.

I need to work on this attitude of living in the moment. Finding joy in the moment. Beauty and perfection and happiness in the as is.

I don't seem to be getting it.

I read and read. And meditate. And love. And stay confused. And sad. And happy. But deep down... numb and sad. What am I doing wrong???? What am I being wrong???? Why does quieting my mind bring up such awful feelings?

3-23-98

Newsweek states raising a child costs $1,455,581.00. How funny. Don't they know— Love is the only currency that counts.

3-25-98

The past two days— Full, wonderful days! I am

Ghostwoman

learning to let go of fear. I'm reading Deepak Chopra's book, *The Path to Love*. Slowly I am learning what faith is. Learning or remembering? It doesn't matter. It's been so long forgotten.

I begin to know this process of understanding also from my Kabbalah class, when I can follow the teacher, that is, and not fall asleep.

The four steps to spiritual awareness.

Doing...
   Feeling...
      Knowing...
         Being...

Takes time.

Then there is the meditation class I am taking at the Ananda church. Pretty similar to what I've been doing myself, but it adds the visualization of light beaming into the third eye. I'm not very good at visualizing. Wish we'd spend more time meditating and less time listening to the teacher talking.

By this time I had finished *Many Lives, Many Masters*, written by Dr. Brian Weiss, a psychiatrist, and was halfway through *The Path To Love: A Guide To Spiritual Self-Healing* by Deepak Chopra, M.D. The first book was an account of a patient whose chronic anxiety was related to past-life traumas. Most importantly, within six months of working with past-life regression, the patient was free of her anxiety for the first time in this life, and stayed that way! The second book was more difficult to grasp, the way Dr. Chopra went on about letting go of everything you want to hold most tightly to. I didn't know about that,

Chapter 4: The Next Three Months

and had a hard time finding the truth in such a statement. I also had difficulty understanding Chopra's concept of how the people in our lives are a reflection of our "Selves." How could others be simply a mirror for the deepest part of who we are? These ideas challenged my understanding of reality, but I had fun chewing on them and hunting for the bit of truth that they held for me; a truth that evolved, and continues to evolve over time.

I was most grateful to have my appointments with Dr. Bice. His non-confrontational attitude allowed me to explore my thoughts and feelings in a supportive atmosphere. He encouraged my curiosity. I didn't have to be right, or even know where I was going with my contemplations.

Soon I found myself wondering if my own bubbling sadness might have a subconscious origin. Perhaps it was past-life related, since there didn't seem to be enough misery in my life to explain the sadness that kept percolating through my meditation. Dr. Bice didn't exactly disagree, though he seemed to find plenty of reasons for my melancholy from what I told him in my sessions about life with Frank. Still, to satisfy my curiosity, he tried a little hypnotherapy with me one day.

He sat in his chair and spoke monotonously while I focused on my breath. This went on for about fifteen minutes and I don't remember that he said anything significant. Then he asked one of my thumbs to identify itself as a "yes" response. My hands rested on my knees, palms up, while I gazed softly beyond them at the carpeted floor. I waited. I breathed deep and easy. And after a while, one thumb raised up. Slowly, very slowly, but clearly it had raised up without my conscious intention. Similarly a "no" finger, my other thumb, presented itself. It was quite a curiosity to me.

This took up most of the hour, but Dr. Bice took the time at the end of the visit to explain to me the theory of what was happening. This technique was engaging my unconscious mind, which was finding expression through the involuntary movement of my muscles. It was the same principle used in muscle energy testing, a technique used in a number of alternative medicine practices. Then Dr. Bice went on to tell me how I could put myself in a relaxed state, ask myself questions, and listen for an answer by observing my thumbs.

That evening I entered my meditation and prepared for the thumb thing. I asked if I needed to go back to some forgotten place, in order to heal completely so that I could give as much as I wanted to give to this world, **and** be happy. I asked if this place was the cause of my sadness. Yes and Yes.

I asked if our old house would sell? Before the summer? Yes and Yes.

I asked if the new house was O.K., and about Frank and our love for each other, and after a few more questions I realized that all my answers were yes answers. Yet, I have never thought of myself as intuitive at all. It was either that, or I needed a hypnotic thumb repairman.

After a while I stopped with the thumbs and relaxed into my more usual meditation. I found myself able to let go of my thoughts a little more easily after having exhausted my questions. I focused on my breath and let go of everything. For a change, I felt a peacefulness that I hadn't felt for the last few days. And I felt a love for myself, just for trying so hard.

He who knows others is wise.
He who knows himself is enlightened.
—Lao Tzu—

Chapter 5
Of God and Madness

The beach house was an auction item I'd "won" at a benefit for the building of our synagogue. The description had said that there were three separate bedrooms plus a loft. Perfect for us and another family, so we invited our closest friends, a family we had known since before we had our children. We planned to rendezvous at the house for the last weekend of spring break. Iyra told me that a vacation with our friends anywhere was better than a vacation without our friends anywhere. Wise daughter, that Iyra.

We packed up Friday morning, a rocky morning. Frank was impatient and directed his anger at me. I hadn't organized things well enough according to him, and as a result we were getting a later start than he desired. His criticisms stung and I withdrew, as was my habit, packing up in silence, avoiding his eyes.

I spoke to Frank as little as possible while he drove us to the coast, and it was early afternoon when we neared the house. I broke my silence to read the directions, and we pulled off the highway and followed

Ghostwoman

the back roads into the quiet little beach community. Four or five blocks of modest houses and a handful of empty lots filled the space between the main road and the sand dunes.

The house didn't look like much from the street. Gray, weather-beaten wood siding with only a couple of small windows on the east side. The simple front door was next to a single garage. There seemed to be a second entrance to our right, up a narrow wooden stairway on the north side, but it was out of view, with the exception of a corner of the first step.

The kids tumbled out of the car and I dug out the key. We entered through a modest, dark basement. It was only for two nights, I thought, as I walked past the laundry room, then up the narrow stairway to the upper level. There, the house opened into a large room with a vaulted ceiling and floor-to-ceiling windows almost covering the far wall. A deck wrapped around the house on the outside. Light poured in as I opened the blinds, letting sunshine fill the delightful space. A broad smile at last took hold of my face, yanking the corners of my mouth up from their doldrums, where I'd been ruminating about the problems between Frank and me.

The loneliness had become unbearable. How long can one live isolated in heart from those one is closest to? A human heart can only contain so many tears.

Jade and Iyra ran up the remaining stairs. "Check out the loft, Mom!" yelled Iyra. "Me and Emily are sleeping here!"

"No, I want to sleep here with Eric!" Jade countered. "Weeee!!!!" he added, jumping on the mattresses that sprawled across the floor.

"Looks like there's plenty of room for all of you, so don't start fighting over it."

The loft was just over the bedrooms, and open to the living room below. Its ceiling was high, with dormers on the sides, and it had a built-in cabinet with bedding supplies and games. I limped around, as jolly and delighted as the kids.

Frank thumped up the stairs with an armload of stuff. "Isn't anyone going to help unload? Come on, you guys!"

What was the rush?

Out we went through the upper sliding glass door and down the steps on the shady side of the house. Frank carried Mondeau, now ten weeks old, down in front of me. He'd heard that puppy hips are sensitive and that they shouldn't be allowed to do stairs for a couple of months. I grasped the railing and limped down the stairs behind them.

After lunch we headed out for a walk to the beach. Frank and the kids went ahead of me, slow as I was with my air cast and wimpy leg. A cold wind and intermittent clouds stole away the warmth of the sun. I climbed over the shallow dunes to where I could watch the waves crashing against the shore, and took a deep breath of cool, salty air. My family was running around with Mondeau. But I, unable to run at all, chilled quickly, and headed back to the house for a cup of tea.

Sitting on the sofa, the sun returned and shone brilliantly through the windows on both sides of me, as if to tell me this was where I belonged. I propped up my leg, and pulled out *The Path to Love*. I was near the end of a chapter titled "Why We Need Passion."

"When passion is gone from a relationship, both partners must be honest in stating that they have desires... The critical step is to eliminate your partner entirely as the cause of the problem and take responsibility for your own feelings...."

Passion... gone from a relationship... I was sharing my life with a man who didn't seem to have a kind word for me in those days, who claimed to love me as long as I remained on my side of the bed. I couldn't touch him, not even a hug, without feeling him tense up. And on the emotional and spiritual levels, things felt even emptier. How could I eliminate Frank entirely as the cause of my problem?

"If you are honest in search of your own feelings, you will hit upon love... You want the return of spirit within you, which is the return of God...."

Paula and kids arrived just before the sun went down. New energy floated in on the fresh ocean air, and I could feel myself lighten up like the spray on the tops of the bridal veils.

I've noticed that when Frank and I are walking on eggshells and the energy between us is all tight and painful, the appearance of a friend, any friend, smoothes the tension. We bury our difficulties for a while and resurrect the pleasantness that we've misplaced. It's not pretend, it's real pleasantness and it feels luscious. We just couldn't seem to find it between the two of us by ourselves anymore.

That first evening, Frank played on his keyboard, the kids played with the puppy and each other, and Paula helped me in the kitchen getting ready for dinner. This was our play, just chatting about this and that in the way that women friends do. It is a way that feels so natural, caring and meaningful, where words just flow like streams into a river. Talking massage therapy.

After dinner Frank whipped through the dishes like he always does, and the kids departed to their game-filled lair. Frank returned to his keyboard, Paula accompanied him on her drums, and I kept rhythm on a little djembe drum for a while. Fun, but not what I needed that night. Soon I returned to my book and contemplations.

Chopra offered a perspective on Love that was different from anything I had ever come across. I was fascinated with the way I understood him to approach relationships as manifestations of "ourSelves," — some higher part of our being that actually includes the other. I had never been introduced to a notion of "the other" as

Chapter 5: Of God and Madness

anything besides a separate entity before. It was confusing, yet I kept trying it, looking at the way I was seeing Frank and me and trying to find it all somewhere inside of myself.

Where did Chopra come up with this stuff?

Paula's husband had to work all day and didn't roll in until late that night. Most of us were asleep by then. I was lying in bed with a heavy feeling in my chest, listening to the distant sound of the ocean, smelling the tart cool saltiness of the night air. The wind had died down, but the rhythm of the sea, dancing with the shore, was an enchanting whisper. I had chosen to forgo my evening meditation so that Frank and I could go to bed together. He crawled beneath the covers and turned his back towards me.

How long was it before I heard the car pull in? The door open and close. Footsteps. The downstairs door open. Footsteps up the stairs, and quiet voices disappear into the night.

3-28
It is a rough night
when the one you love
to wrap your arms around
and into your heart,
turns
the other way
without acknowledging your love.
Tears flow
as quietly as they are able
not wanting to disturb
your cocoon of
Detachment
is not love.
I cry

Ghostwoman

and try to look beyond the tears
and hold up a mirror that somehow
shows me myself
And God
Our relationship gone array.
Finally understanding...
how painful non-acceptance is,
I did not understand,
still have trouble
accepting, allowing, and loving
when what you are doing is hurting me.
Perhaps, but I don't know,
this is the ebb before the flow.
Understanding does that,
Opens the blocks and allows the spirit to soar.
Must it continue to allow pain in?
Understanding has its time, and its need.
Will happen when it is ready. When we are ready.
Pain has purpose.
Always.
Faith.

It was another beautiful day today. The sky was still clear and sunny, and the breeze strong, but not quite so cold. The weather reminded me that I'd forgotten our kite back at home, and the breezes so wanted a toy to play with.

Went into town for a kite. I needed something to lighten my spirit. Jade and Iyra came with me. I didn't even know if the town had a kite shop but I was in the mood for a little adventure and Paula

Chapter 5: Of God and Madness

was in the mood for ice cream. Found a great kite shop. Colorful nylon hung from the ceiling, lined shelves, and filled canisters. Birds and bats and dragons, geometric shapes trailing colorful tails arched over the doorways.

I planned to come away with one kite of my own choosing, for a change. The perfect one for the strength of the breezes that day, a simple kite, an inexpensive one. Like walking into a gourmet chocolate shop and expecting to walk away with a 33-cent candy bar.

Iyra chose a beautiful rainbow box kite, Jade chose a two-handed stunt bat. It was too much fun to compromise. They were so happy!

Of course, then they wanted to do the flying when we were back at the beach. Paula and I had fun just walking and talking. I was telling her about Chopra's book, and thoroughly enjoying sharing what I was reading with someone who appreciated it and didn't always have to challenge whatever I said.

My shin and ankle throb. I pushed it a bit. I walked about half an hour! Lovely beach.

Spent much of my walk rehearsing. I'm afraid I won't be able to get out what's inside me. It just goes round and round inside my head and it has to come out. I have looked at all the options.

I love him very much. I thank him for being. I can handle the distance everywhere but in bed. It's not the lack of sex, but the lack of any closeness, any sense of being loved. I don't know why it feels so unbearable, it just does.

So I need to be by myself.

We're responsible for our own happiness, and for changing our situation to change our unhappiness.

I'll move into the basement.

A cloudless night with a delicate cool breeze. I got up my nerve and asked Frank to go on a walk with me after dinner. The kids and Mondeau were all happy as puppies playing together, and Paula was content to hang out with them.

We headed down the outer stairway. I wanted to hold Frank's hand, wanted him to want to hold my hand, but gripped the railing and slowly stepped down the stairs behind him. He waited for me at the edge of the road in the darkness.

Then we walked toward the ocean. We talked. Rather, I talked. Told him I couldn't take the distance between us anymore. I couldn't handle what felt like such indifference and coldness. I needed to feel loved.

By the time we were headed back towards the house, we were at it again about all the same old birth control shit, ending with him needing to keep his distance—physically and emotionally.

For all the times we'd been over this, I could still feel my rage ignite with his words. Seven years of birth control pills with all the unpleasant side effects that only I had to experience. The IUD that wouldn't stay in, and all those wretched instruments only I had to endure. I almost choked on my anger but kept it in check as we lingered outside at the foot of the stairs.

"Then I'll move into the basement," I said.

"Forget it! We might as well not be married!" he answered.

"Fine!" I exploded, unable to control my feelings anymore. "Then I'll just have to leave! Because I can't take it the way things have been!!"

Chapter 5: Of God and Madness

My words ended in uncontrollable sobs, and I turned as quickly as I could and bolted, limping, up the stairs past our friends, and collapsed on the floor of our darkened bedroom. I wedged myself between the far wall and my side of the bed, and sat there on the floor, hugging my knees to my chest, grieving in convulsions of tears.

Frank followed me into the room and closed the door behind him. He sat on the edge of the bed, saying something, trying to console me as best as he could. He told me that he'd put the IUD in.

"You believe that your excellent oral surgery skills allow you to do better than my gynecologist with her years of experience?" I could not understand this man. I could not understand his way of seeing things. What seemed practical to him felt like a pompous ego to me, and I resented it! "How would you feel if something happened?"

"I'd be careful. Nothing would happen." Then he went on about how any skilled surgeon could watch a video. "I've done hundreds of procedures."

"Why can't you hear what I need for a change? What feels right to me? It's MY body. I'm tired of being with a man who can't honor what feels right to ME! Just go away! Leave me alone!"

And he left.

And I allowed myself to keep crying, and to shed tears for all those moments of sadness and denial and all the loneliness I have felt with Frank and in my life.

Such tears feel endless when they begin, as though they come from a sea and need to be gotten rid of drop by drop. But when I gave myself permission to empty the sea, it dried up. I was tired of crying, tired of being sad. I was ready to leave my tears and move on.

Sitting no way in particular, I shifted my focus from my grief onto my breathing. There was nothing left for me to want to think about. There were no solutions that would bring me anything but pain, no good options. I put my attention on the in and out of my breath. The movement of my belly, soft belly, allowing the breath to flow fully. Feeling the movement inside of my nose, I focused only on my breath and blew the pain away.

I cannot say for sure whether I added a mantra with my breathing that night or not. I was experimenting with a little bit of this and that. Sometimes when I meditated, I'd breathe *yod, hay, vav, hay*, the mystical Hebrew letters signifying the nameless name of God, the God beyond all names. Sometimes I'd breathe *hong sau*, as taught in the Ananda meditation class that I'd just begun, visualizing a beam of white light entering my head between my eyebrows. Sometimes I'd just breathe *let go*. But sometimes I would simply and totally focus all my attention on all the nuances of breath. Soft breath. *Neshamah*, the Jewish word for breath and soul.

Then it happened. In just a few breaths, the breath of a solitary human became one with the One. My separate consciousness merged with the ocean of consciousness that is All. And it was all One. God.

My awareness moved from being a grieving woman whose marriage was breaking up, and feeling connected to nothing but my own misery, to being connected and a part of Everything! Not just in thought, but in my very being. I was One. I became consciousness, as if it was my skin and all that it contained. Only I wasn't conscious of anything in particular, just my own being.

I felt this experience as surely as I know the sensations of pleasure and pain, the sensation of touch. Yet this was beyond a sensing. I was in a place where my senses no longer existed and all I experienced was Knowing, Being, and the purest of Love that was beyond my imagination or remembered experiences.

Though I had read about unity, until now it had been little more than a beautiful concept. It was the core of my religion. *Shema Yisrael, Adonai Eloheinu, Adonai Echad.* God is One. I always loved this concept, but that was all it had

Chapter 5: Of God and Madness

been to me, an idea. This was beyond idea, it was experience. The difference between looking at a picture of the sea, and swimming in and merging with it. And yet, I was still separate enough to experience this wonder as myself. Distinct, yet part of a seamless existence. I vacillated between these realities in a rhythm not unlike breath, in, and out, I was One with the One, and self, and One.

I struggle over words. How can one describe wearing consciousness? And the feeling of absolute Love? Love was simply poured into me and filled me with such fullness and such indescribable Joy! I was enveloped! Saturated! Breathing Love! Breathing Oneness! Or had I stopped breathing? Just being was all that mattered. Being *was* Love. Being *in* Love. Loving Being!

Can one describe the feeling of love in hopes of conveying the feeling itself? It's like trying to describe color to one who knows only black and white. Words can never explain that, only experience can define some things. And then we say, "OH!!!! That's what it is! NOW I understand!"

We chatted that night, God and I, my thumbs twitching wildly. Yes and no to all the questions I could think to ask of God. My God. That found the time to make itself known to me. My God. Who cares deeply and loves me more than I'd ever known love before. My God. Who was Love. Pure Love. And was pure consciousness at the same time. My God. That wasn't a spark within all matter, but of what all matter was a part of.

My thoughts drifted back to my home circumstances. Without words, I came to understand my problems with Frank as issues whose answers lay buried more deeply than we were ready to know. I felt a profound love for Frank and fully accepted where he was at this time. I felt so completely loved myself that I was in need of nothing. In one breath, I went from feeling like I had no choice for happiness in my life but to leave Frank, to wanting to

Ghostwoman

marry him again just so I could love him!
What about past lives? I asked. "Who have I been? Has my history added to my fears? My insecurities? My heavy heart? Did I die in the Holocaust?

No particular answers came to my questions, only the awareness of the lack of separateness between any of the individuals my mind tried to dwell on. We were all lives. All people. We were the ten million people executed by Hitler's brokenness. We were Hitler, Hitler's mother. In unity consciousness we were all lives. All people. One eternal Being. And in that wholeness, we were pure Love. It didn't make any sense. I didn't have any answers that could tie the discrepancies neatly together. My questions were not so wise.

Soon my questions of separateness were peeled away by my desire to simply bask in the sensations of Absolute Love. Nothing else mattered in the depth of such Love. All that mattered was Love. And the questions of separateness became like specks of dust on the ocean. My rational thoughts, my drive to understand the order and logic of all things, melted into the Sea.

At some point I climbed out from behind the bed, and into it. There I lay, experiencing this miracle, listening to the sounds coming from the other room— decisions to cut into the chocolate cake I'd baked for everyone for our weekend together, light conversation and laughter, the music of the children's voices.

Frank came to bed sometime that night. He lay on his side, and for the first time in months, I was at peace with it, needing nothing to be different from the way it was. I needed nothing from anyone, only others to whom to give.

The following morning I was back to being my separate self, though somehow very different. Emerging from the bedroom after my morning meditation, I felt a blush of embarrassment, being such a private person and having been somewhat hysterical in front of my friends as

Chapter 5: Of God and Madness

I dashed by them the night before. But their smiles, their warmth, were more beautiful than ever, and I was so delighted they were with us.

"Good morning," I smiled. "God, it's another gorgeous day!" We passed our hugs around and prepared pancakes together, waking the kids with the aroma. After breakfast we all headed down to the beach for the last time before heading home.

It was always beautiful at the coast, but that morning everything was particularly crisp and perfect. The wind had died down to a perfect kite-flying breeze. We took turns without quibbling, enjoying the kites no matter whose turn it was to fly them, dancing with the kite shadows on the sand as though we, too, were flying. I picked up a stick and dragged it behind me, drawing large swirling designs in the damp sand. Sometimes I'd pause and begin the swirl in the opposite direction, creating crests, like the waves, in a sea of swirling and curling lines.

Mondeau and the kids played chicken with the waves. Iyra and Emily kept a close eye on Mondeau, quickly scooping her up when a larger wave caught her by surprise. Frank threw her sticks, which she knew how to retrieve with as sharp an instinct as she had for nursing, then he retired to the top rocks of the jetty and spent some time gazing out into the ocean.

"What are you drawing, Mom?" asked Jade.

"I have no idea, but isn't it cool?" My masterpiece was expanding over a huge area. Footprints dotted the background and the waves erased the lower reaches. "Here." I handed Jade my stick. "Have a go at it for a while."

I sat back on the warm sand and read more of *The Path To Love*. I believed, and still believe, that the knowledge that Chopra shared helped propel me into the state of universal consciousness. I had been practicing a new paradigm for how to love. How to honor *myself*. How to love myself. How to love God by honoring *my* feelings and desires. Loving by accepting, rather than controlling. And at the same time, somehow trying to see the others in my life as a reflection of myself, honoring them as well. Dr. Chopra helped me to let go of judging, helped me to look at things beyond the bad and the good, denying nothing, seeking truth, always.

During our drive home I breathed contentment. Absorbing the scenery as it passed by filled me with great joy and love for the earth. Everything looked more alive. The colors of the tall fir trees through the mountain pass were more vivid, the landscape more three-dimensional, and even the sounds emanating from the radio, more clear. For the first time I could ever remember, I was able to distinguish the words of the songs that played, not just the repeated chorus and the melody. It was a striking difference and quite remarkable. I was awake!

Frank eventually became weary while driving and I took over for the last bit. It was nice to feel the familiarity of our established road-trip pattern, and to have the chance to drive my family quietly along while they all slept. I felt the comforting hum of the engine, and the gentle massage of the tires on the road.

I loved just being.

Chapter 6
On Being, Madness?
and Creating a Mess

Over the next two weeks, the mechanics of my life went on as usual. I'd wake the kids and drive them to school, go to work, attend to all the details of home life, i.e. shopping, cleaning, meals, laundry, after school activities, music lessons, miscellaneous commitments, etc., etc. The nuts and bolts of my days were no different.

What was vastly different, however, was that the ghostwoman disappeared!

I wore all my flesh those days! My emotions were alive and full and spontaneous! They danced with an immediacy, responding as One to the events of my life. They were free, floating, and felt as natural as breath, as the wind, as the storms and the sunshine. And the most prominent of these emotions was a state of joyfulness that was fuller than I had ever known. Its depth came not only from the happiness that I encountered, but in the fullness of my being, whether I was happy or not.

Distinct physical sensations also accompanied me

during this time. Mentally I felt high, sort of dizzy, but not the fall down dizzy, the light as a feather kind of dizzy. And I had energy like I hadn't experienced for decades, since before the mononucleosis of my late teens. None of these new physical sensations felt bad, but they were alien to me and I had no one to ask about them. They made me a bit nervous, so I stopped meditating for a week or so, thinking that perhaps my head would settle down more quickly that way.

But my health in general amazed me. I walked with barely a limp, quite an improvement from the days before when I'd just stopped wearing my air cast and was walking with much instability and weakness. And there was also a spontaneous improvement in my flexibility, pathetic after six months of relative immobility. All bodily functions flowed perfectly. Even my dry skin felt supple and moist, where it had been dry and itchy for years.

In addition to the emotional, physical, and energetic healing, there was also a different quality of thought that I expanded into. My mind often danced with insights that were so new to me that it was clear they were not my own. These thoughts were similar to the "aha" sort of thoughts of creative inspiration, only they were louder and more vivid than my usual thinking. There was an intensity to these thoughts that was stronger than my everyday small mind. It was more of a knowing than a thinking.

Sometimes this knowing was assisted by my unrelenting questions and the responses of my twitching thumbs. But sometimes ideas and understanding just filled me. Abstract ideas shifted from an intellectual process to an experiential one. I was dipping into a bottomless pot of consciousness soup and ladling out bites from the hearty stuff at the bottom.

Knowing that I am embraced by Love at all times.
Knowing what Appreciation and Gratitude *feel* like.
Knowing that all things go as God's will.

Chapter 6: On Being, Madness?

Knowing that everything has a purpose, which ultimately directs us back to knowing God, ourSelves, and Love at its fullest!

At no time, however, did I feel like had all the answers. On the contrary, every answer I received simply filled me with more and more questions. Paradoxically, being filled with knowing made me feel like I knew less and less every day.

Words. I became aware of the powerful meaning of the subtlety of language. Every language was holy, not just Hebrew, Sanskrit, and Latin. Puns, homonyms, they were all rooted in meaning. I also became aware that words had a creative power of their own just by being thought, spoken, and written.

Words, those little bundles of differentiated consciousness, **mattered**. In every sense of the word. Matter: to make a difference. Matter: substance with form. Somehow words created both.

Experiencing this thought from a place beyond my imagination, gave it an authenticity that cemented these ideas into something firmer than belief. It felt absolute, even when contradicted by my rational thinking.

I played with these new thoughts, but they would soon cause me trouble as I clumsily tried to incorporate my budding understandings into my medical practice.

I continued to do the holistic counseling that I'd begun before the mystical experience. Only now, the spiritual aspects were even more important to me. Emerging from the place where all matter and spirit are One, I sought these connections in most of my patients, trying to get at their problems from a place where the deepest and most lasting healing could be accomplished.

One patient, an African-American gentleman about sixty-five years old, looked at me deeply and told me it felt good to have a doctor that talked about God.

Two other patients, both younger people struggling with drug addiction problems, also shared how much they appreciated my perspective.

"It's so nice to have a doctor that listens to you and recommends a book instead of a pill," one young man said as he left.

Unfortunately, not all of my patients appreciated the spiritual perspective I was sharing (though I did not share it with all, only with those for whom I felt it appropriate, and especially when I saw it as potentially central to the patient's healing). One woman about my age, a new patient, came in complaining of pain in her foot that sounded like *plantar fasciitis*, a common disorder I'd diagnosed many times before. This was a recurrence for her, and she did not want to take any anti-inflammatory medicines, the usual first line of therapy for this problem, though not a particularly effective one. Not being a practitioner who did cortisone injections, I had little else to offer her besides counseling on appropriate shoes and a referral for the injections.

"What do you think I should do?" she asked.

"I could refer you to a podiatrist," I responded. Then I sincerely added, "But I believe one can get this sort of problem from trying too hard to stand on your own two feet. One needs a certain balance in these matters. Perhaps you need to let other people help you, let God give you a hand."

The patient became quite upset at these words, and immediately began putting on her shoes. She couldn't get them on fast enough. Again, I offered her an appointment with a podiatrist, but she was clearly not interested in anything else I had to say.

Feeling terrible about having made this poor woman feel worse than she felt at the onset of her visit, I retreated to my office to collect myself. I realized I was talking too directly about God, and was expressing unproven causation. Yet why didn't she just brush off my suggestion? Why was she so deeply affected? I decided to adjust my approach and limit my spiritual counseling,

Chapter 6: On Being, Madness?

focusing on where the patient was coming from, and adding psychospiritual connections sparingly. From there I could assess how the information was accepted. Besides, it felt like the meaning of an illness had the greatest healing capacity when coming from the patient, not from me. Perhaps my job was simply to help my patients discover their own truth.

I quickly sat down at my desk and wrote an apology to the foot patient, then let it go. These new perspectives on disease were too inspiring to linger on a minor mistake of how to share them. I enjoyed having the new approaches for my chronic patients. These were the patients most appropriate for psychospiritual counseling, and they were the ones who seemed most appreciative of it.

While charting, I reflected back on my readings from Chopra's book, in particular, the focus on following my heart's desire to remain connected with God. Was it really in my best interest to chart the way I'd like to chart?

Thumb twitched wildly, "YES!" So with nervousness and excitement, I adjusted my descriptions a bit. I let go of the sterile observations of patients and added some heartfelt subjective observations in their place. I let go of all the tedious writing that I felt was unnecessary, but was required as protection against possible litigation. Defensive charting, no need for that now; I was in loving hands! I worked quickly, was out on time, and thoroughly enjoyed myself!

I am nearing the end of Chopra's book.
"...Enlightenment requires total honesty with yourself and others, regarding both emotions and actions. -
The ego keeps you from being honest - thinking that it can control its destiny... all our fears have already happened."
April 1st.

Ghostwoman

A full day of work.

A good day.

Knowing God. Consulting with God.

Allowing the day.

Learning from all.

Sharing love. Acceptance.

Seeing a part of myself reflected in everyone and everything, all of us being mirrors.

Jade and Iyra teach me. Jade with his, "Don't talk God with me." And Iyra, "I don't need to meditate. I don't think it would help me. I'm glad it helps you. I don't have anything I need to meditate about."

Thank you.

We were sitting down to dinner at our old wooden kitchen table. Mondeau dutifully lay down by Frank's chair. He'd taught her not to beg, but to just lie down while we ate. Iyra kept eying our "Oh, isn't she just the cutest!" puppy. She had already begun teaching Mondeau a few tricks. Jade updated Frank about the science museum I'd taken him to after school, while I finished putting the food on the table.

"I had a great day today," I said as I sat down. "Went over to Sue's this morning for that massage she wanted to give me once my cast came off. I never did get the massage. We had too much fun just talking about life and God and Spirit and all that stuff. She is sooooo wonderful! Has a bunch of books on metaphysical philosophies and healing. Gave me a whole box of those Chinese patches for Iyra's growing pains." Then I started talking about how pain is needed for spiritual growth.

It seemed so clear to me by this time, that my spiritual experience was the result of the profound

Chapter 6: On Being, Madness?

emotional pain that I'd experienced over the preceding months. Without it, I would never have allowed myself to open up in total surrender. Pain was forcing me to look deeper into myself than I had ever had the need to do before. And in looking deeply, I was looking into God as well. Who needed God when all was going smoothly?

Frank became upset and angry with my comments on the need for pain.

His anger was met with my own, fiercely defending my beliefs. My voice began to rise. I spoke with conviction! And then, a fleeting thought came to me. A thought whose content is long gone, but what remains is the memory that it was an amusing thought. And my ferocity changed, just like that, into laughter.

Perhaps it was a pun that set me off. Puns were flying through my head those days. In my ordinary state of consciousness I was rarely quick enough or alive enough to catch them, but during this time, words swam in puns.

Frank stared at me with a look of total perplexity. He was not used to me laughing with such fullness and intensity, nor with getting angry, nor with letting go of anything so quickly. "What's wrong with you?"

"Nothing," I said, reeling in my laughter. It was contagious and the kids were laughing by this time, too. They're usually the ones who laugh all the time over little things. "I'm just feeling great!"

At some point we resumed our conversation on pain.

"You want growth through pain?" Frank asked loudly, as I began clearing the table and walked over to the sink. "I can show you pain. Hey kids, your mom wants pain!"

"No one <u>wants</u> pain!" I responded back. "You're missing the point. The point isn't to hurt each other. There's a difference between intentional pain. Intention is what matters, always to have good intentions in your heart!

"Now I have a meeting to go to. Good-bye." With that, I stomped out of the room, grabbed my keys and was out the door.

I left my anger behind me. Attached to nothing, I was happy just to be feeling. I acknowledged what I felt, then let it go.

...the message is always through pain and pleasure. It has to be. Because the message is always through feelings.

Being in touch with feelings is the key to understanding God. And it's always easier when you share your pain. Share your feelings. This is the key.

Feelings. People who know, share their feelings with you. It's that simple. But you have to share them all. The good ones, and the frightening ones, and the pitiful ones, the ones that feel so embarrassing.

The people we love give us just what we need to understand. Asking. And Allowing. This is Love. And I'm writing my story because if I don't write it down, I'll forget. Until... You know... How beautiful God is.

Thank you for showing me the meaning of gratitude.

WOW.

Every little message along the way helps.

April 4th. A night I must have amused God greatly.
Dreaming.
A tremendous throbbing headache. I had not had such a headache in a long time. I was told in this dream

Chapter 6: On Being, Madness?

that the only way to get rid of my headache was to call my Rabbi and have him bless me with my Hebrew name. I woke up.

My head was throbbing.

2:30 am. And I am the sort of person who feels guilty calling anyone after 9 pm. "Do you want me to call Rabbi Avram, now???"

My "yes" thumb twitched.

"Can't I just take some Advil?"

Right thumb twitched, "No."

I slowly pulled myself out of bed, and quietly stepped down the stairs to the kitchen. I fumbled around in an old cabinet to find our synagogue directory, watching myself with disbelief at what I was about to do.

"Hello, Rabbi Avram? This is Harriet. I'm very sorry to awaken you at this hour, but I have this terrible headache, and I just had a dream, and in my dream I had a terrible headache, and God let me know that all I needed was for you to give me a blessing on my head with my Hebrew name, and my headache would go away."

Rabbi Avram was kind and uncritical of my invasion of his sleep at this most ridiculous hour for a headache. He asked me a question.

"No, I don't know what my Hebrew name is."

Then he asked who I was named after, and I told him my grandfather, Harry. He asked if I could tell him anything about him, but all I knew was that he was my father's father, an optometrist, and that he died of a heart attack before I was born. Avram told me he'd have to know more in order to know my Hebrew name. Then he told me to get back to him when I had more information. I thanked him for his time, and apologized again for awakening him in the middle of the night.

While we were talking, my headache eased up. But shortly after I hung up, the intense throbbing began again. "You want me to call my mother now, and find out something about my grandfather?!?"

Ghostwoman

A "yes" twitch. At least it was six a.m. in Florida, where Mom and Dad live. Without any argument this time, I called. "Hello, Mom? Sorry to call you so early in the morning."

For some reason, Mom was already awake, and she was so delighted to hear from me that we didn't even mention the oddity of the time.

We had a wonderfully sweet and peaceful conversation, talking unhurriedly about who I was named after. It turned out that I was not named for my father's father after all, but for Harry Cabot, my mother's grandfather.

As my mother began to tell me about Harry Cabot, she realized how much we had in common. He, too, liked to spend time hiking in the woods. And he hunted for wild mushrooms, as I had done for years. He could tell if they were edible by tasting them. He'd put them on the tip of his tongue and spit them out, a dangerous practice I had heard of only once before. It was the same technique used by my first love, who introduced me to wild mushrooms.

Mom went on to tell me that my great-grandfather was not an educated man, having been an immigrant who needed to work, but she remembered him to be an extremely loving man and very wise.

"And one other thing," Mom remarked. "He would only let your Bubby have two children. Even back then he was aware of the problem of population. Your Bubby wanted more children, but he was insistent that they keep their family small."

This last piece of information sent my skin tingling. Mom didn't know about my abortion, and I wasn't ready yet to share this. Our conversation was gentle and soft, and I wanted to remember it that way. But I did manage to ask her if she was concerned about my visits to the gynecologist.

"No, not particularly," she answered.

Chapter 6: On Being, Madness?

"Good. Because it was nothing serious. And I didn't want you worrying, what with Nana having died of ovarian cancer, and all."

This had been on my mind since recently, when I'd *felt* the truth that we somehow create new reality through thought. In what way I didn't quite know, yet it felt deeply true. And yet, as I rolled this thought around in my head, I could certainly see the many instances when this was not the case. I wondered, what was the context in which this truth was true?

Over the next few years (and counting), I would continue to try to untangle this knot of confusion. I encountered vast amounts of literature on this subject, and met new friends who lived their lives based on this principle. Thought. Prayer. Research showing the efficacy of the mind effecting healing and altering matter. The implications were riveting! Meditations on peace. Meditations on healing. Thought *IS* a form of action. But how much versus how much physical action? Was thought just a catalyst? Concepts in quantum physics supported the blending of object and observer. Oneness. So much to meditate on, so much to play with.

Talking to my mother that night, I was quite simply relieved that there was no chance of any illness in the making through any conscious worry on the part of Mom or myself.

Mom's comment about my great-grandfather being a wise man jolted me back to an old forgotten memory of my childhood. It was a clear evening, and the first star was out. I looked between the thick leaves of the avocado tree outside my bedroom window and made a wish. I wished for wisdom.

We hesitantly said our goodbyes, each of us lingering over this unusual morning conversation. My headache was down a couple of notches. Then we hung up, and back it came.

"You want me to call Rabbi Avram again???!!!???" I

can't do that! He's likely to have just fallen back asleep!"
Throb. Throb. Throb.

My thumb twitched "yes."

"Excuse me, Rabbi Avram?... Yes, I know what time it is, and I'm very sorry to wake you up again. You said to call you back when I found out more about Harry, and I have, and I still have this awful headache. Please, could you just imagine your hands on my head, and say the Hebrew word for wisdom for me?"

"Chochma. Chochma. Chochma," I heard the tired voice repeat over the phone.

"Thank you. And again, I'm very sorry to have awakened you. Good night."

My headache was a little better, but not yet gone. "Chochma," I said to myself, and was filled with the sound of the name of Frank's grandmother.

Oma.

"You want me to call Oma? She's so old. It's too late. I can't do that to her."

I called Oma. Luckily, her answering machine was on, and I didn't awaken her. "Hi Oma, it's Harriet. I just wanted to tell you that I love you."

My head was still hurting as my cold body crawled back between the covers. Jade had crawled in bed with us. I laid a hand on his and Frank's heads and whispered a blessing, "May you be the bright and joyful, creative, star that you are, for your whole life. And may you have the opportunity and find the joy in sharing your gifts with others."

My head still hurt.

I nudged Frank awake. "Will you put your hands on my head and say 'Chochma' three times?"

He obliged me without question, then rolled back over to go to sleep.

Still my head hurt too much and I meandered back downstairs to snuggle more upright on the sofa. I continued my conversation with God, watching the

Chapter 6: On Being, Madness?

twitching of my thumbs. That they twitched without my intention, that I was a part of the collective oneness that I understand to be the Oneness of God, that my twitching thumbs gave this collective wisdom the opportunity to chat with me— that was enough. I could live with a little headache.

I awoke later that morning. My headache was gone.

It was an Aikido morning for the children. I remembered Sensei would be having some people filming the class that day, so I hurried the kids to be on time, insisting that Jade put on a clean shirt.

"I'll bring the puppy with us," I said. Then, after consulting my thumbs, I consciously, and nervously, left the leash behind. Mondeau was only 10 weeks old and very lively. But I was practicing letting go, and feeling a faith so deep and complete that all I felt I needed to do was observe and listen, and follow the moment, and all would be as it should be.

The Dojo was quite full. The usual half dozen children had expanded to twelve, and there were many visiting adult observers. A tall tripod holding the video camera stood proudly in the center of the viewing area, surrounded by a small sea of onlookers. The space was almost full, quite unlike our usual sleepy gathering.

As usual, Sensei's large black Lab was tied to the desk by a short leash. Mondeau, tucked snugly in my arms, eyed the big dog.

"Why didn't you bring the leash, mom?" asked Jade.

"You can't just let her run around all over the place. You need to put her in the car!" added Iyra, freaking out about my letting go.

"It'll be O.K."

She rolled her eyes. Still looking concerned, she and Jade headed for the mat to bow in.

All the seats were taken, so I found a place on the carpeted floor between Sensei's dog and the tripod. Mondeau squirmed to get loose from my hold, so I relaxed my grip, knowing that I could grab her if the need arose. She wriggled free, then stepped mischievously up to the big old Labrador.

Mondeau, the petite, blond, golden retriever.
The Lab was big and black.
Mondeau the free.
The Lab was confined.

Mondeau began running circles around the Lab. I just wanted to grab her and get out of there, but I kept feeling and remembering, "Let go. Let go."

The onlookers' attention shifted from the warm up exercises the class had just begun, to the dog action happening in the back. Sensei, too, became slightly distracted. Mondeau jumped into the arms of a beautiful young Asian woman sitting near by. She laughed hysterically as we realized that Mondeau was trying to nurse her through her clothing before squirming to go free.

She ran up to the mat, but not onto it. She looked back at me. She ran back to me, then back again to the edge of the mat, this time placing one paw timidly on it before looking back. It wasn't long before she took the plunge and ran around on the edge of the mat. She was like a child testing her limits.

Sensei cringed, then said very quietly, "I just don't want her to pee on the mat." The cue that I'd been waiting for. I smiled and nodded to Sensei, then lovingly whisked Mondeau into my arms. We retreated quietly down the steps and out onto the sidewalk below.

I breathed a sigh of fresh air briefly, then realized that I now had the street to be concerned with, as Mondeau wriggled desperately to be free from my arms again. I wanted to hold even more tightly, but remembered Chopra's words of letting go. What do we let go of? That which we would hold onto most tightly.

I was not sure that this was what Chopra was talking about, but there were not many cars on this part of the

Chapter 6: On Being, Madness?

road at 9:30 on a Saturday morning. With some trepidation, and an eye up the empty road, I allowed my puppy her freedom.

Amazingly, at ten weeks, she came when I called her. She explored the bits of grass surrounding the parking lot, content to not wander off. She never stepped a paw into or even near the street.

I sat on the edge of a planter filled with green grass. It was elevated from the level of the sidewalk and quite comfortable. The sun was out. The sky was the bluest of blue and my puppy happily bounced from one interesting smell to the next.

Across the street I noticed three people walking up the sidewalk, headed our way. At first, they appeared to be passing by on the other side, and would not come close to us. But just as they were about to cross the main road to the opposite side, the woman caught sight of Mondeau. "Look, a puppy!" she smiled, and pulled her two companions in a different direction to check out Mondeau.

The people were dirty, appeared to be leaning on one another, and smelled of alcohol. They wore big, warm, smiles. The eyes of the woman and one of the men were kind and gentle. Those two looked clearly Native American, with their broad faces and straight black hair. Though unkempt, I found them to be very beautiful. They seemed to be trying to take care of their friend. He, too, had a big smile as he observed Mondeau. His eyes were a beady combination of sparkling and somewhat hazed over. There was something about him that I didn't trust.

Mondeau thought they all smelled quite magnificent. She ran over to them, wagged her tail and little body furiously, and peed on the sidewalk. We all erupted in laughter.

"She's a golden retriever, isn't she?" the woman commented.

"I had a golden retriever many years ago," said the

Native American man. "She was just wonderful. Her name was Cookie."

"How funny," I chuckled. "That was my mother's nickname for me."

"My name is Red Dog," said the woman.

"We met two adorable red dogs just last weekend, two Irish setter puppies. They were wild about Mondeau."

"I'm a bit worried that I don't have her on a leash right now," I continued. "But I'm trying to let her be as free as she can be." A look of understanding reflected in the eyes of my acquaintants. "We have one pet who we can't set free, yet. It's a garter snake we found up in the mountains four years ago. I found him with my son, who I keep trying to convince to let the snake go, but he hasn't been ready to do that. He's afraid Jerry will die in the wild after all his terrarium-bound years. That's our snake's name, Jerry."

The second man's name was Jerry. We all laughed again. Jerry the snake.

"We used to have a snake that went free in our house," said Red Dog. "It kept all the rats and mice under control. Maybe Jerry could be freed, do the same thing for your family?"

How could I tell her we didn't have any mice? "Our Jerry is about the size of a fat pen. I'm afraid he'd be eaten by Mondeau long before he found anything to eat."

We agreed Jerry was better off in his cage for now. Then these pleasant people were ready to move on.

After shaking hands, Red Dog asked if I happened to have any spare change. I rummaged around in my wallet, and finding very little change, added my lucky Susan B. Anthony dollars to the meager collection. I gave this to Red Dog, wishing it were more. "Do you need anything else?" I asked.

She smiled warmly again, her eyes shining their gratitude. "No, thank you, the change will do just fine."

Chapter 6: On Being, Madness?

We wished each other well, and they wobbled on down the road.

Aikido class was just about over. It was time to go home. The kids were somewhat humored, somewhat mortified by Mondeau having caused a little distraction at the beginning of their class.

"Nothing bad happened. I was right there waiting for a signal that I needed to do something."

"Like when she was running all over the place!" said Iyra.

"Was she hurting anybody? She was just making a lot of people laugh. When Sensei asked, I took her outside. What's the big deal?"

"You didn't have a leash! She could have gotten hit by a car!"

"But she wasn't, was she? I kept an eye on the traffic. And besides, I believe that all things that are meant to be, will be. I mean, heck, I was hit by a car while standing in the bakery!" Then I paused before sharing the rest of my irrational rationale. "Besides, my thumbs told me that Mondeau would be safe."

"What do you mean your thumbs told you?"

"Well, my thumbs seem to twitch yes and no. It's something that I learned from a visit with my therapist one day. One thumb twitches if the answer is yes, and the other thumb twitches if the answer is no. I asked if Mondeau would be safe."

"How do you know your thumbs are always right?" asked Jade.

"I don't. But they seem to be right so far." I knew better than to get into a discussion of the unity awareness I'd experienced and wholeheartedly believed in, and how that was connected to the thumb thing. I let it go.

Then the kids let go of worrying as they settled into the back seat of the car, basking in the warm tongue kisses of their puppy.

That afternoon I brought Iyra and Jade to Shabbat School, where I began to set up for the class I was scheduled to teach. Nothing like teaching a somewhat disinterested group of eleven-year-olds something that they think they already know, while you're in the middle of an experience of non-ordinary consciousness.

I focused on feelings, the link to knowing, which our society most profoundly smothers or misunderstands.

"How do you *feel* about Passover? What *pleasant* feelings do you have about Pesach? Any bad feelings?" I drew a yin-yang symbol on the board and talked about how everything has pleasure and pain. Everything that we come to know, we come to know by both sides of the experience.

They began their answers with, "I think..."

"No!" I cried, my arms waving wildly about, animated by my own excitement. "I want you to feel, not think for a change!!!"

After a slow start the conversation became quite lively. Hands sprouted and waved in the classroom air like branches on a blustery fall day. Comments became enthusiastic.

"The horseradish really burns your nose. That doesn't feel too good," said one boy.

"And I'm hungry! The whole time we're doing the service I'm starving and the food cooking smells sooo good it just makes me hungrier!" said another.

Another voice, "And I hate it when you've just learned the four questions really good, and you don't get to say them because a younger kid gets to say them."

"Those are all things that feel bad," I remarked, noticing that the negative was being remembered before the positive. "What about positive feelings?"

Another pause to think about feeling, then the hands started waving again.

"I love the feeling of all the family being together and getting out the really special dishes and making the table

Chapter 6: On Being, Madness?

look so beautiful," said one of the girls.

"I love the taste of the *charosets*!"

"I like the way it feels to find the *affikomen*."

"I hate the way it feels when someone else finds the *affikomen*."

Then I added my two cents. "I hate the way I feel when I see *all* the sad faces of the children who didn't find the *affikomen*. So at our Seder, the person that finds it first gets to hide it again. Then we keep doing that until everyone gets a chance to find it and win a prize."

My ten-minute introduction to Pesach had stretched into twenty and had to be cut off so we could have time for my teaching partner's presentation and my ending focus on slavery.

The mood was so spontaneous that my partner ditched his prepared presentation on rituals, and continued drawing out the material from the students. Then I moved in with my slavery discussion. I'd been enjoying thinking about this and had looked forward to sharing the modern day plight of the farm workers and some new legislation I'd been opposing that would make the workers little better than slaves.

Slavery. What did it mean? Who was a slave? I could have spoken at length about this subject but restrained myself, remembering an old Jewish folk saying I'd found in Ann Landers, "We have two ears and one mouth so that we can listen twice as much as we speak."

Shema Yisrael.

Shema.

Listen.

At the end of the class, one of the girls, Sara, blurted out, "I liked that class. It made me feel so close to God!"

Frank had been busy in the garden all day while the kids and I were out and about.

Driving up our driveway, I left the pleasant day behind and shifted gears. Car gears, teacher gears, into wife gears, mother gears. The kids tumbled out of the car, then ran off to find their puppy, whom we'd left with Frank for the afternoon, wondering if she missed them while they were gone.

I walked the long way into the kitchen, around the house, curious to see what was opening up in the yard. The thick corner of bulbs had become a blooming mass of yellow daffodils and blue hyacinths. A few of the early rhodies had unfolded. The ivy hadn't composted yet, what a mountain! Only Frank could have the vision to see it composted (in two years time it would grow the biggest and sweetest squashes I'd ever tasted).

There was Frank, crouched down and pulling weeds. A large collection was filling up the black garden bucket by his side, dandelions and morning glories, mostly. He'd freed the wild violets, and the small patches glowed in vibrant shades of purple.

"How's it going?" I asked.

"Still a lot more weeds to go, but I'm making some headway."

"It looks better all the time. And now you get to garden surrounded by flowers instead of traffic! See you in a bit, I have to fix dinner." And I continued around the house, beyond the raised beds, up onto the old deck with its few rotting boards, and into the kitchen.

It was a pleasant meal, but as we neared the end, the kids told Frank about my morning escapade at the Dojo.

"Why didn't you use the leash, Harriet? That was really stupid!"

Once again I tried to explain about fate, about my thumbs, trusting the universe, letting go, plus there was hardly any traffic. But I might as well have been talking to the moon.

"I can't believe you, Harriet. You talk like we have no control over anything! We do have control. Use your head!"

"Sometimes we have control and sometimes we

Chapter 6: On Being, Madness?

don't. Sometimes we need control, and sometimes it's O.K. to let go. That's all I'm saying. But since it makes you all too uncomfortable, I'll use the leash from now on."

I stood up and began clearing the table and putting away the food.

"Do you want Mondeau to be killed?" Frank blasted at me.

"Of course not! Look, you don't understand, that's O.K. I said I'd use the leash from now on!"

But the badgering continued. All three could not let go of it.

"Would you guys get off of my case!" I yelled, slamming the ladle into the pot I was about to wash. I darted out of the kitchen, through the dining and living room and up the stairs, collapsing onto my bed where I cried.

Sad, mad, misunderstood, I couldn't ever remember being so upset at my family. I was usually so emotionally passive, afraid to show anger, afraid to have such a feeling.

Iyra came up after a while. I was still crying, and she put her little face next to mine, telling me, "It's O.K., Daddy's just afraid something will happen to Mondeau. He just told us a story about a dog that ran into the street in front of him once, and he ran over and killed it. He still feels awful about it."

"Thanks for coming up and trying to help me feel better. That was nice. I really appreciate it." I smiled through my tears at her beautiful face. "And thanks for telling me Daddy's story. I'll be fine, I just want to be alone for a while." We hugged, then I kissed her before she went back downstairs.

Two weeks of letting go. Two weeks of not being embarrassed to feel, or to show my feelings. Two weeks of feeling humor instead of humiliation.

Early on in my visits with Dr. Bice we talked about fear. What was I afraid of? At first it was survival, but spiritual understanding put that fear somewhat to rest, though not quite to sleep. Then new fears crept in, fear of embarrassment, rejection, and loss. These were trickier fears to abolish. How delightful it was to live two weeks with such fears at a minimum. Being myself, completely.

Frank and I had one more good little argument during this time. We were standing in the middle of our office, my piles of papers and opened and unopened mail merging so intimately on my desk that the surface was completely hidden.

"You always interrupt me!" he claimed.

"You go on and on and by the time you're done saying what you've got to say, I've totally forgotten what I wanted to respond to at the beginning of your monologue," I retorted.

Frank resumed talking by the paragraph, if not the page.

"There you go again," I stated.

"You interrupted me again."

"You paused," I countered. "I know, how about I raise my hand when I desperately want to comment about something you just said before you say much more and I lose my thought?"

"Harriet, I'm not in school! I'm not raising my hand."

"Then I've had enough of this conversation because it's just making me angry and I don't want to be angry!"

I turned on my heels and left our office, resuming the kitchen cleanup that Frank had begun.

A loud **THUNK** could be heard from the other room. Within a few moments, Frank sheepishly emerged into the kitchen.

"You're going to hate me," he said softly.

"I'm not going to hate you. What did you do?"

Putting down the kitchen towel, I walked back into the office to see what terrible sort of unforgivable thing this lovable man had done. I'd been working on the bills and pile on my desk, and had a bag filled with paper

Chapter 6: On Being, Madness?

recycling on the floor by my chair. Frank had turned the bag upside down on my still unfinished desk of papers.

I returned to the kitchen, where Frank was still standing. "Looks like you got a little angry yourself," I said. "But I don't hate you. You finish up the kitchen. I'll go tend to my desk."

What a mess.

I began sifting through the papers, one by one, a tedious task I had no mind to do. Is there anything there I need to be concerned with? My thumb twitched "no." And into the paper recycling bag went all of it! The organizations wanting money would surely write me again. Most of the bills were paid, perhaps all; they'd let me know otherwise.

Then I saw what had made the loud thunk. A fist-sized hole was gaping in the wall to my right. I don't know why, but it made me laugh. He's such a beautiful, strong man!

I covered up the hole the following week with a *Happy Anniversary* card that arrived in the mail from my parents.

Chapter 7
Settling Down

Sunday, April fifth. A beautiful spring morning, perfect for the old friends that were coming up for a visit that afternoon with their children.

"Mom, I need a bathing suit," Iyra informed me.

"Well, it's Sunday, the stores don't open for a while. How about we head out after breakfast and get there when they open?"

There was no hesitation. No agonizing over wanting to make sure I had everything I needed for our lunch, or whether there was still going to be time to pick up the house. I was listening to the day ask me what it needed and delighted to be able to accommodate it. I was so accustomed to filling my day with being completely responsible, that letting go, completely, was all it took to stoke the fires of my joy. Iyra hopped up and down when I told her we could go. She loved to shop, and she did need a bathing suit.

We chatted like two birds in the car together, laughing and talking. But we arrived at the store, twenty-five minutes away, only to discover that they were closed on Sundays.

Chapter 7: Settling Down

"Could we please try the mall?" Iyra begged.

The mall? I hadn't enjoyed malls for years. The crowds, the bombardment of stuff. I asked my thumbs if they could give me a hand. Emphatically, they twitched, Yes! So off we went to the mall, guided by my thumbs.

Fifteen minutes later, confronted with the unpleasant task of finding a parking space on the weekend, I asked my thumbs for some assistance. They wiggled yes, then seemed to wiggle left and right. I followed the cues through the crowded lot to an open spot just in front of the entrance to a store I hadn't intended on going into. But hey, why not?

We walked through the housewares department, looking at all the pretty stuff. Beautiful glass atomizers with little glass humming birds on top of them caught my eye. On sale! Mother's Day was coming up and I thought of Eve and Oma.

I bought the little gifts, then walked Iyra to her clothing section. She liked being on her own, so I left her looking through the bathing-suit sale racks. From there I wandered through the rest of the store, my thumbs leading the way. It was wild. I merely supplied the transportation and paid the bills. My thumbs led me to a tee shirt with Frank's initials on it. To socks, which he needed. To ridiculous boxer shorts for my dad with a big picture of Scooby-Doo for Father's Day. To some remarkable skin cream for my mother and I, with vitamin C, ginkgo, and ginseng. Shorts and a sweater for Jade. Cologne for myself with the name of *Eternity*, some for Frank with the name *Obsession*, and another one for the two of us with the name *One*.

"Where to next?" I asked without speaking. And from there I was led to the juniors department.

In my state of unconditional love, I had metamorphosed from thinking I needed to somehow separate from Frank, to wanting to remarry him for our anniversary the following year. It would be our 13th. I was looking for a dress for the wedding renewal ceremony I had been envisioning. My fingers did the shopping. I wasn't in the mood to agonize over clothing. I walked slowly. My thumbs twitched "yes" and "no" in front of the racks of dresses. I fingered through them leaving my thumbs free to tell me when to stop. They picked out a shimmery long purple dress with spaghetti straps. Originally over a hundred dollars, it was marked down to just under half of that. I did not try it on, my thumbs assuring me it was unnecessary, and I was delighted to find the dress marked down further to fifteen dollars! My God loves sales!

Iyra, too, had found more than she was looking for, and like my experience, all were bargains from the sale racks that we could not pass up. We bought them, and with a tremendous sense of lighthearted joy, headed quickly back home where our guests had already arrived.

Sunshine mingled with beer and juice. Laughter and smiles danced with the freshness of the April air. Iyra and Lishka cut armloads of fragrant japonica bells, camellias, rhodies and daffodils. Every vase we owned was soon overflowing with the fluorescent energy of spring. The boys rode skateboards down the inclined driveway while wary fathers (whose own younger daring had taken each of them close to death) stood back and observed.

Loree and I moved inside to fix dinner, where I noticed I was having trouble reading the recipe. This made me think about the way antidepressants and other psychoactive drugs can sometimes cause blurred vision, and I wondered whether a similar chemical reaction had occurred in my brain spontaneously. But this was of no consequence, as I had few of the called-for ingredients anyway. I improvised with great delight, and found the result quite pleasing, though Frank told me they were the worst lentils he'd ever eaten.

That night, after our friends had left and I was still enjoying the lingering taste of friendship, I received a call

Chapter 7: Settling Down

from my clinic manager, Theresa.

A few of my patients, three to be exact, had complained about the spiritual counseling I'd given them. One nurse had also voiced a concern about me. Theresa was calling to tell me that my clinical supervisor, Betsy, wanted to talk to me and go over the complaints that upcoming Tuesday.

A wave of concern washed over me. Then a wave of reassurance. Everything has a purpose. Everything would work out just as it needed to be.

Monday, the sixth. At work I continued finding great satisfaction with my patients. I was seeing the divinity in every one of them. I'd been charting it too. 'Beautiful soul with sparkling eyes,' replaced my more usual mundane observations of their size, sex, and ethnicity.

I was careful to record what I felt were all the important physical findings, but left out charting my observations when I felt them to be inconsequential, which was quite different from my usual tendency to be compulsively complete. Another major change since my spiritual opening was that I began charting my spiritual counseling for the first time, though I had been working with it for months. I wanted to record what I was doing in order to follow the outcomes of my new counseling strategies and the breath meditation that I was teaching. Would it be helpful to teach patients how to meditate in a short visit? Would they follow through? Meditation was documented to be beneficial. But would it work to teach it in this manner?

I let my charting flow. I even signed a couple charts, "Love, Dr. Cohen."

Tuesday the seventh.

Betsy and I met in a conference room in the corner of the administration area of the clinic. It was a large, plain room with no windows. Inexpensive boardroom tables

Ghostwoman

were arranged in a rectangle, surrounded by chairs.

Betsy was sitting with papers and charts in front of her when I arrived, her bifocals resting delicately on the edge of her nose. She turned and stood up, greeting me with a warm, but restrained smile.

We sat down and Betsy shared the complaints. One of the patients was the foot woman, who I was well aware of and feeling a bit embarrassed about. The other two took me by surprise. The first was a new patient to me, who came in complaining of a sinus problem from allergies. She felt that I implied that her allergies were a creation of her own mind, a view that she could not endorse.

She thought it wonderful that I'd found my spirituality but thought I was pushing it to the extreme. She did not plan on continuing to see me. I had prescribed appropriate medications for her at the end of her visit.

But it *is* all a creation of our mind, I thought to myself. It's just that the mind is so much more than we are aware of, than we understand it to be. It's so much more than our conscious thoughts. Many months later I would attend a lecture and read various studies linking the allergic process to our thoughts and emotions. The lecturer almost quoted my own intuitive understanding exactly. But I did not have such documentation at the time that I spoke with this patient, or with Betsy. Nor would it have mattered.

Betsy also brought up my chart notes. "Your objective component includes the statement, 'Very kind and considerate young woman... beautiful smile. Expressive face.' And your plan includes the statement, 'Lovely discussion regarding the true nature of all illness.'"

Perhaps I overestimated her kindness and consideration, I thought whimsically.

"The next complaint came to one of the nurses. The patient complained of religious overtones of her visit with you, and the prescription of herbal remedies."

We looked through the chart together and I

Chapter 7: Settling Down

remembered the patient well. Again, I had never seen her before, as she was a patient of another physician I worked with, who was not in the office that day. She was a difficult patient with chronic complaints of total body pain, and was there that day in tears from her agony. On methadone treatment for heroine addiction, she'd failed all conventional western therapies for her pain, including tricyclic antidepressants.

"Review of your chart notes reveals a brief description of the patient's subjective complaints. Under Objective the note reads: 'Severe pain in total body. Very tearful and painful.' The assessment reads, 'Discussed issues of love of self. Patient unable to forgive herself for how she raised her children with her drug abuse.' The plan is, 'demonstrated breathing exercises and explained how to forgive. Rx Detox tea TID. Discussed accepting love and how to look at life to accept wisdom. Pt open to discussion. God Bless.'"

I guess she wasn't as open to the discussion as I thought. Perhaps it was the tea recommendation, which I'd given her as a meager attempt at detoxification. I knew little else to specifically recommend, but was learning from my Ayurvedic studies that detoxification would be of therapeutic benefit. I remember her concern that there might be something in the tea, which would turn her urine test positive. If she had a positive urine test, they wouldn't give her the methadone. "I doubt it will affect your urine," I'd said to her. "But if it did, perhaps you might consider it a sign that it's time to get off of your methadone."

The fourth complaint was also a difficult chronic pain patient who was on maximal medications and wanting more. Again, I had run out of conventional options. With this patient, I thought I remembered speaking to her over the phone, but I had not recorded the conversation in my usual, fastidious manner.

The last issue was about my charting on an alcoholic patient I had known for years. I had discovered for the

Ghostwoman

first time that he was a Vietnam Vet who couldn't forgive himself for all the people that he'd killed in the war. I had discussed looking at his life in a way that gave his experiences meaning and value. Again I'd talked about the value of forgiveness. It had been a beautiful visit. The patient hadn't complained. Why had the lab tech felt compelled to make an issue of my charting these things?

"Betsy, I thoroughly agree I was off with some of my assessments and my approaches. The foot patient gave me clear feedback when I saw her that I was coming on too strong with the spiritual connection to illness, and I've already backed off significantly. I realized that one has to approach patients from where they are coming from."

"I'm glad that you agree," she said. "You also need to return to more conventional charting, and I don't want you doing anymore religious counseling."

"Wait a minute," I objected. "First of all, what I've been sharing is spiritual counseling. I haven't mentioned any particular religion. On the contrary, I've supported whatever religion my patients practice. Secondly, I agree that some of my counseling was inappropriate, but I've been using spiritual counseling with many of my long term patients for the past three months, and they've given me positive feedback. Also, there's research that supports the integration of spiritual counseling and meditation for numerous chronic illnesses, including chronic pain."

Betsy paused for a moment while looking at me. "What I can do is talk with some of the ethicists and gather opinions from other physicians about the place for spiritual counseling as a therapeutic option. But for now, I do not want you to raise this as an option for your patients, and do not offer spiritual explanations for their problems."

"I can agree to hold off for now, but let me know when you meet with those ethicists, because I think we're withholding valuable strategies for many, although not all of our patients."

Chapter 7: Settling Down

Betsy put down her pen and took off her glasses. "When did you get so interested in all this spirituality stuff?"

I paused, and began slowly, a little nervous, but also relieved to be invited to share my experiences. "It started with the accident. I was going through a lot right then, far more than the accident. I started seeing a therapist who told me about Caroline Myss' work, and it just resonated with me. From there I picked up one book after another, all written by western-trained physicians, supporting the integration of spirituality for healing.

"Then I started meditating, and found it so helpful that I began teaching my patients how to do it. Have you heard of Herbert Benson? He's the head of the hypertension clinic at Harvard and has a couple books out about meditation.

"Everything was going smoothly until the weekend before last, when I had the most amazing experience!"

I could feel my face light up as I told Betsy about my unitive experience and how I'd been feeling since then. I told her about my thumbs, about unity consciousness, about our being connected to God, "And I've been sort of high since then and have this wonderful energy! I didn't even need as much sleep as I normally do the first couple of nights. I wonder if it's anything like mania?"

Betsy sat up, leaned back in her chair, and reminded me not to do any more spiritual counseling with patients until she spoke with the ethicists.

One night I had a mildly prophetic dream about a very dear friend of mine. In my dream, I was visiting her in a post-op surgical room. She had just had a tumor removed and was reassuring me that she was going to be fine, that they had gotten the whole thing out. In the dream, it was her uterus. "How did you know you had the cancer?" I asked. My friend was sitting up on her stretcher with her hospital gown draped modestly around her.

"I'd been losing weight and Mom nudged me to have a check up."

It was so real, so vivid, so unlike my usual absurd dreams. I called her the following morning to ask about her weight. She lives three thousand miles away and I hadn't seen her for over a year.

"Fine," she reassured me. "Perhaps I've even put on a pound or two. Why?"

I told her my dream.

"Nope. I'm up to date on all my gynecologic check ups and I feel great!"

Two months later she would give me a call. Found a breast lump. It was small, and they got the whole thing, but it was malignant.

All of these experiences were miraculous to me, but there was more. There were two more messages that I received in the night. They came during states that were not dreams, but were not normal waking either. The first was about consciousness, that consciousness was energy. It had power. It was not just a thought that needed some physical action to follow, but at some level it was some kind of energy in its own right. I had never heard or read about consciousness in this way before, and it would be years before I discovered there was a whole field of healing research on this concept that had been quietly taking place for decades.

The second awareness was not trumpeted in with any particular importance, but just melted in one night with all the other goings on. I had started it with a question, wondering if there were other people who had experiences like I was having, or was I alone? I remember being answered with my thumbs, then playing more than, less than, to get some idea of how many people had had such an experience. There were thousands of us scattered across the globe. And there would be more and more, all the time.

Chapter 7: Settling Down

We are entering a messianic age, an age of consciousness expansion. An age of compassion, gratitude, and healing. An age of peace.

What did that mean? I asked. Will we be done with war? Would the people of this earth stop needing to endure any more Holocausts? Bosnias? Vietnams? Tiannaman Squares? African tribal massacres? Tibetan tragedies? AIDS epidemics? What about....? and What about...?

To these questions I received no answers, just the reminder *To live in the moment, To trust God, To love all people, and To love the earth.*

Aside from my boss, I told few people directly about this unusual state of mind that I'd stumbled into, but I did make an appointment to talk to my Rabbi. I felt badly about having called him in the middle of the night and wanted to explain myself.

We met in a coffee shop, and as I began to tell of my mystical experience, he looked around nervously at the other patrons and suggested we take a walk. We ambled through the old neighborhood, and by the time we returned to the center of the village where we'd begun, he advised me to study the connection between spirituality and healing before using it in my practice. He also suggested that on a personal level, perhaps I needed to go back to understand where my experience had come from.

This was very good advice, but my mind jumped to the thought of past lives right then, and flashed to my childhood dream of the torture chamber. I was a wall and could feel all the vibrations of the screams. "I don't think so, Rabbi. Anymore, I get a cold chill at the sight of someone else's blood. I can't even do simple procedures without my hands shaking violently. No thanks, I'm not going back there!"

Looking back, I doubt that my Rabbi was talking anything about past lives, but I was reading about such things, and so it was on my mind.

Ghostwoman

"I've got to get back to work," Rabbi Avram said to me. We smiled, said our goodbyes, and turned and went our separate ways.

I didn't feel badly about my conversation with Avram. He'd let me share my story, and that felt wonderful. I thought I was talking to someone who could understand me. But things changed after that conversation. Where he'd previously been very warm and inviting, always engaging me in conversation when we'd meet at Shabbat School, he began to keep his distance, never pausing to say more than a polite hello, rarely even meeting eye-to-eye. Soon afterwards, a friend told me he'd approached her and told her he was worried about me. And he never brought up my experience again, or asked me how things were going with my work.

I wanted so terribly to share what I'd experienced with someone who could understand. I wanted to share that joy with another soul. I hadn't told Frank everything, just a bit here and there, as he was not one to talk about God, but I had no one else to turn to. One morning I walked into our office, where he was catching up on his paper work. I stood in the doorway, smiling, feeling the excitement of perhaps connecting with him about this precious experience.

"Do you know?" I asked, wondering if he had ever experienced unitive consciousness.

"Know what?" he asked without looking up from his work.

And I tried to ask him, and tell him about the loss of ego.

"Harriet," he turned to look at me. "We need the ego. It tells us what to do, what's right and wrong. It's who we are."

So, I shook my head in agreement. He was right, too. And left him to his paperwork, and went back to the Passover Seder preparations I was attending to before I'd interrupted him.

Chapter 7: Settling Down

I worked two more days in the clinic, then spent the next week at an internal medicine conference. Betsy was also there, and we sat next to each other during a few lectures, privately sharing our opinions and sometimes confusion over the material presented. On the last day of the conference, she sat down with me at a far corner of the lunchroom.

She leaned toward me over the small table between us. "I was very concerned after the conversation we had last week. I need to let you know that I've consulted with the attorneys for the county, and I can't let you return to work until you've been evaluated by a psychiatrist. You'll be placed on an administrative leave of absence until I get a report that you're O.K. You'll be paid during this time."

I was stunned. I knew when I began my unusual charting that things could get interesting, but I didn't think it would happen so fast.

Yet I could understand Betsy's position. My state of mind was most non-ordinary, though I hardly felt it as pathological. "I can certainly see where you're coming from, and why you need me to see someone. I've been seeing a psychologist for the past six months and have an appointment with him next week. He's a Ph.D. I can have him send you a report."

"No, it needs to be a psychiatrist," she said.

"Well... then I think I should at least see someone familiar with spiritual experiences," I suggested.

"I need you to see someone of *my* choosing," she answered.

At first I balked, though perhaps not out loud, knowing the probable illegality of such a request and my vulnerability with the wrong psychiatrist. However, I trusted Betsy's intentions to be in the best interest of both myself and my patients, so I decided to let go, to let the will of the Divine guide the choice. I agreed to see the physician of her choice, whoever would satisfy her insecurities, as I was intrigued by my experience and had nothing to hide.

With the time off I could start the yoga class I hadn't had time to begin. My broken leg had grown strong enough to try something besides swimming, but it was still only half the size of my "good" leg. Frank's wrist was healing from the carpal tunnel surgery, and he would be returning to work in a couple days. With me at home, Mondeau wouldn't have to stay alone outside in the pen all day. She was still a puppy, and I hated having to put her out for such a long time. Also, there would be more time to read. I was impatient to dive into the book I'd just picked up, *Healing Words* by Larry Dossey, M.D. It looked like it would have the documentation I needed to validate some of my opinions and counseling strategies.

Then there was the other book that had almost jumped off the shelf at me when I'd picked up Dossey's book. It was written by psychiatrist, Dr. Dennis Gersten. *Are You Getting Enlightened or Losing Your Mind?* I skimmed it, then put it back on the shelf. It wasn't going anywhere and I had enough to read. Perhaps now I'd have time for that one as well.

Within days I received a memo from Betsy summarizing the patient complaints and concerns, the issues that this raised for my job with the county, and her recommendation on how to deal with it all. The memo went on to state her concern that I was neglecting the allopathic approach in order to introduce a spiritual perspective into the encounter.

The reality is that with chronic patients and fifteen-minute visits, one must always pick and choose what, in particular, one thinks is best to help a patient on any one day. With all the literature I had been reading about the efficacy of treating illness from a holistic perspective, and the reality that mind and spirit issues had never been deeply addressed with these patients, I felt that along with appropriate allopathic care, these other aspects of health

Chapter 7: Settling Down

needed to be integrated into their treatment plan.

I was also reprimanded for advocating a therapeutic approach, which had not been endorsed by the agency. And lastly, my somewhat unusual and sometimes incomplete charting was addressed in the traditional terms, not in the light of what I understood the power of the written word to be while in this altered state. Liability fodder, as opposed to intentional, creative energy. Betsy included my agreement to resume charting in a more conventional manner.

4-28

Outside the air is amazingly warm. There is a lovely breeze this morning. Taking Mondeau out last night, bare feet, in just my flannel nightgown. I was cool but not chilled, a pleasant surprise. It will be another cloudless, rainless day today. I wonder if the haze will be as thick? The distant hills disappeared yesterday afternoon.

I look outside my den window and smile. The apple blossoms have opened! The lilacs are in bloom. Azaleas of apricot strut their flowers, vincas still adorn the ground in purple stars. Trillium, bleeding hearts, and rhodies— the pale yellow one outside the dining room and kitchen window glows. Toward the fence, the rhodies Frank brought from the other house are red, and becoming pink. The last fragrant white camellias linger below the tree house.

Our Clareodendron have sprouted and are looking healthy and vigorous. The rhodies planted between them are blooming. Roses growing, snow peas up, strawberries, garlic, and potatoes happening. The blueberry bushes are flowering and the raspberries are

Ghostwoman

growing from their severely pruned nubbins.

    The dogwoods are coming alive. We have three of them, all different. One has leafed out, one is still sleeping and one has a few flower buds. They all looked so beautiful and fiery red last fall, one of the rare beauties I was able to appreciate about this house in my somber state of mind. Below them the potentilla and yellow tulips color the lower canopy of bushes, perfect complements to the blue vinca and delicate violets at their knees and toes. Those pretty pink little bells are blooming, too. Debra told me they're called Coral bells.

    The front slope, where Frank has torn out the ivy and replanted it with rhodies and trees from the old house, is awakening. Our pineapple quince and apple tree survived the transplant and are doing well. The pines are showing new growth, so very appreciative of the loving gardener who freed them from their ivy chains. Nearby, tulips of pink and deep, almost black-purple bloom above a sea of hyacinths. The monarda is coming back, peonies popping out with buds all over! And the garden in front of the basement, it too is lovely, rhodies opening up, albino bleeding hearts open, ground cover colorful and dotted with wild strawberries throughout.

    Hard to believe all I could see last fall were weed trees. There is a large old bay tree with a knobby trunk near the house in the back, and in the corner of the property grows a walnut tree about forty years old. It's a youngster compared to the ancient walnut that graced the back yard of our neighbors'

Chapter 7: Settling Down

property at the old house. I couldn't bear to watch it get cut down, an inevitability when the property is developed as planned. It's comforting to be the caretakers of such a magnificent tree in our own yard.

The walnut tree has a tree house. I can't get near it, as it requires rather skillful maneuvering through and up the laurels and camellias under the canopy of the tree. Frank and the kids have no trouble and enjoy climbing into it. They tell me it's safe. The previous owner called it a liability.

Even those weed trees on the side of the house, which looked so moth eaten by the end of the summer, look beautiful this time of year. Currants, cherries, birch, and hazelnut, their blossoms are delicate and sweet.

I hope my appointment is fruitful today. I've agreed to give the IUD one more try. I no longer worry about the outcome. I'm looking forward, in fact, to my undisturbed waiting room opportunity to read. Which of the books that I am reading should I bring? I am like a student again, studying so many at one time.

Tomorrow's appointment with the psychiatrist, Dr. Eugene, has been postponed a day. I do hope I can return to work next week. My thumbs tell me two weeks— not next week. What a waste of county money and time. However long it takes, I will delight in my own happenings, but am concerned about my patients. I'm sure they'll do fine. I just care about them and miss them.

Chapter 8
Evaluation #1

My heart pounded madly, as if trying to escape from my chest, as I entered the converted Victorian house. It lacked any names of physicians on the outside of the building, which added to the mystery of Dr. Eugene, the psychiatrist I was told to meet at this address. I was not given a phone number for the office, but was told to call my boss if I needed to cancel my appointment for any reason. There was something about this arrangement that made me feel wary, but I decided it was not worth my effort to address it for the time being. I left myself in God's hands.

The entryway opened up to a small waiting area where a young woman sat behind a glass window. Yes, I was in the right place, and Dr. Eugene would be with me in the conference room shortly. I sat down only briefly before being led to a fairly large room with a long boardroom table in the middle. Dr. Eugene sat on the opposite side of the table from where I entered. Behind him was a wall of windows allowing me to look out upon a small central courtyard built of brick. It was filled with a

Chapter 8: Evaluation #1

few dormant trees, and sunlight filtered through large windows making the whole scene quite lovely and tranquil. After brief introductions I sat down facing Dr. Eugene.

He was a smallish man with a neatly trimmed gray beard that matched his gray suit. He had fine features. His shoulders were a little hunched, but he was otherwise unremarkable. He told me this was an evaluation, not a usual office visit, and as such I could not ask him questions, but could only answer the questions he posed to me. I did ask how long the evaluation would take, as I'd parked in a metered space and had children to pick up from school in two hours. "Shouldn't be a problem," he answered. He didn't expect the interview to take longer than about an hour and a half.

Dr. Eugene asked me all the usual questions about family, childhood, personal history, both physical and mental, then started in on my experience. My answers were straightforward, though I avoided bringing up the details of my abortion. I simply said that at the time, I was going through quite a bit of personal difficulty which I'd worked through with my therapist. Then I moved to my meditative experience.

I was delighted to have the chance to talk with an interested ear about my two weeks. Perhaps, I thought, he will be able to offer some useful insight, for which I would have been most grateful. My western and Jewish upbringing gave me no context for understanding my experience, and though it did not in any way feel pathological, I was not quite sure what to do with it, particularly as it related to Frank and me.

I interrupted the interview at one point. I was not wearing a watch, and there was not a clock in the room. "Could you tell me the time?"

"Two forty-five."

The kids needed to be picked up in fifteen minutes and my meter had just run out. "How much longer will this take?" I asked.

"Not more than five to ten minutes at the most," he reassured me.

Wanting to get it over with and get back to work, I excused myself and quickly put another quarter in the meter. Five minutes later I interrupted the interview again. "It doesn't look like we're going to be finished anytime soon. I really can't be any later picking up my daughter and her carpool from school. I'm going to need to reschedule to finish up."

Dr. Eugene sighed with what felt like a touch of frustration, then we scheduled an appointment the following week to complete the evaluation.

I didn't worry about my meeting with Dr. Eugene. It seemed to have gone well enough.

May 1, May Day!

Today's a cooler morning. Yesterday's temperature felt like 90!! Reminds me, I should go turn off the fans that have been blowing on the kids all night.

It is so lovely in my office with the view of the blossoming trees. Mondeau putters around in the yard while Frank attacks the plugged drain with a snake. He is so deliberate, capable, and has such confidence. He is fearless with projects of the home & garden. Problems or inspirations, he gets things done and seems to enjoy the challenge. Me, I'd call the plumber.

May 2

a mother's life
is tricky.
I count the blessings of my beautiful healthy family,

Chapter 8: Evaluation #1

and still, find myself wanting
mySelf.
lost in years of interruptions and caring for others
so much out there. Needing. Asking and not asking.
But children always ask,
don't stop.
Ask the same thing half a dozen times until I
remind them
I am no more intelligent nor wise than the first
time I was asked.
Often, more than one asks at one time.
Sometimes three
talk to me
at the same time
of different things wanting me to listen
to validate, to answer, to share their space with
my attention and opinion.
Recently it dawned on me that some days I had no
opinion left
besides, close the door behind you please,
I don't like a house full of flies.
I wait and play my music when no one is around
to be bothered.
No one but the unwashed dishes,
the unmade lunch,
the piles of clean clothes you washed this time.
Thank you.
We seem to take turns being dear.
I write,
enjoying words and soft thoughts briefly
until children come in

Ghostwoman

and barrage me with their questions
and opinions, and loud energy, and this is my job
the only job I ever truly wanted
way back when I thought I knew myself.

May 6.

    I have the gift of emotion these days. My heart rides its own tides. I wonder if they mirror those of the sea? Or have I my own rhythms unconnected to anything I am aware of? I, who not so long ago knew what it felt like to feel one with the oneness of all, feel aloneness once again.

    I cycle through opposites and accept this motor that propels me. I live with highs and the lows as long as I can use them both to create. My creativity comes from feelings. I surrender to them all.

    I wonder if others, too, fluctuate in their experience of moods? Those of us who allow ourselves to feel, can we feel otherwise? I remember my days when I was unable to open up to feelings. I wish such detachment and numbness, such isolation, on no one. I wish a life of connection, and reconnection, and awareness of our profound interconnections!

    Requires feeling, the ups and the downs.

    I suppose my second meeting with Dr. Eugene this morning, finishing up his evaluation of me, might have something to do with the heaviness I feel today. The ten minutes it was supposed to take turned into an hour. I have no idea what his impression of my experience is. The interview seemed

Chapter 8: Evaluation #1

to go OK. I was honest, and explained my story clearly. He was polite, but offered nothing.

I feel so alone.

About a week after I saw Dr. Eugene for the remainder of my psychiatric evaluation, I had an appointment with Dr. Bice. I shared what had gone on since my last visit three weeks earlier, and he seemed quite distressed about the unfolding events, and particularly about my work situation.

"Harriet, you may need to get an attorney to work with you. I'd recommend you get in touch with one as soon as possible."

Dr. Bice said he'd call with the name of an attorney he'd met at a conference who had seemed spiritually minded. I thanked him, quietly hoping it would be unnecessary.

May 14

I'm excited with the peace that meditation brings, allowing me to feel the peace in all things. I wanted to share this with Frank. I guess I was explaining how different sitting meditation is from other meditation. He had been sharing that his weed pulling was meditation for him.

"Don't criticize me for what I do if it works for me."

His tone was sharp. His words bit like unexpected red ants. I hadn't criticized him. Caught off guard, my instinct was to flee. I was running late and appreciated this perfect time to go.

A short reprieve. Errands finished, I am once again home, avoiding him. His eyes. Avoiding talking to him— though I think this is what ought to be,

Ghostwoman

to work it out.

    I think he is so sensitive to criticism that he senses it even when there is none.

    I am remembering the perspective I learned from Chopra, my projections and judgments— a reflection of myself? The part of me that, too, is so sensitive to criticism and judgment that I tell my husband very little of what my heart feels. I tell everyone else (that I know won't criticize me!) My safe friendships, my dear friendships. And my journal. And my therapist.

    Today, this festering old wound reopens and I am reminded of our mutual issue with criticism. We have some things in common after all.

It had been a month since I'd seen patients and there was no end to my leave in sight. Clearly my thumbs weren't able to give me any assistance with the timing, or didn't want to. They had twitched "yes" to my asking if I'd be back to work within two weeks, but at two weeks, all I'd accomplished was two thirds of an evaluation by a psychiatrist. A friend, Ruby, who had been developing her psychic healing abilities told me that she could never get any useful answers about time from the spirit world. She'd learned to quit asking.

    I could see a purpose to this limitation. It required the development of patience. I'd been informed of the importance of this virtue during my two weeks of altered consciousness. That was why I'd become a doctor, to learn patience. Patients. Patience.

    Ha! Ha! It was so funny at the time.

    As time passed, my thumbs seemed to be off more and more. At first, I thought it was because the further away I became from my unitive experience, the less

Chapter 8: Evaluation #1

connected my individual consciousness was to Oneness, and the less ability I had to tap into the knowledge that the One has at its fingertips. But I also considered that perhaps I was using my thumbs for the wrong reasons. Before my experience, I was working on being in the moment and accepting that which is, with an open heart. Now, wasn't I using my connection to try to navigate the future? Trying to feel the comfort of certainty when the point is to learn to feel comfort with uncertainty? Or perhaps my twitching thumbs could not give correct answers because "correctness" is a rational process, and the thumb twitching was an intuitive one, I mused.

The rational and the intuitive. How did they fit together? We are born into humanity with two equal sides of a brain. The intuitive right side shares equal space with the rational left. But the rational brain had long since become stale to me and put me to sleep. This new intuitive experience had felt so alive, so vibrant and exhilarating! It taught me the feeling of profound connectedness. Rational thinking had never allowed me to feel such a precious sense of belonging. We cannot rationalize the feeling of Love.

This was paradoxical. Rational thought was shared thought, collective agreement. Intuitive process was the wholly internal and personal process. Yet intuitive perception could touch the interconnectedness of all being.

The rational without intuitive feeling was empty and meaningless. Perhaps in the same way, without the rational follow-up, without the validation of a collective shared experience, intuition would become lonely, isolating, and meaningless as well. Both sides of the brain were needed. Balance is the key.

So I continued to observe, even more closely, where and when my thumbs gave me straight answers and where they didn't. But I could not give them up. The fact that they twitched involuntarily to my questions kept me feeling connected when nothing else did.

I returned to my heart for my guidance, my Jewish heart, though it would be a couple of years before I began to understand my strong connection to Judaism.

In Hebrew, the word for heart is *lev*. Different from the English word, the Hebrew heart is understood as the source of both feelings **and** intellect, intuition **and** rational thought. Similarly, in Chinese and Japanese culture, there is only one character, one word, for heart/mind.

This was the place that I was submerged so completely during the mystical experience: the sea of consciousness that was simultaneously an ocean of love. This heartmind was the place that I returned to for my guidance (though nowhere near the degree of unity I felt during the mystical experience). I listened to my deepest feelings, listened to the clearest thoughts that I could hear, and listened to the feelings that were generated by the thoughts, feeling my way to truth.

Friday afternoon I was in the kitchen fixing dinner when Betsy called. She'd received the report from Dr. Eugene and wanted to schedule a time to get together with me to review it. The soonest time possible was Monday.

Her voice felt cool and distant as we scheduled our meeting, and this made me nervous.

"What was Dr. Eugene's assessment?" I asked.

"We can talk about it on Monday," Betsy answered. "I think you should see the full report."

"And I will see it on Monday, but I'd like to know his diagnosis. I'll do better over the weekend if I know."

"He concluded you had a manic episode," she said.

Frank was standing by the kitchen as I hung up the phone. "It's bullshit!" I exclaimed, after telling him the diagnosis. "I've treated enough manics to know one, and what I experienced was not a manic episode! Some of the features were similar, but my experience and mental

Chapter 8: Evaluation #1

illness are very different. How could a professional come to such a conclusion?" I stormed through the kitchen space looking for things to clean and put away, trying to regain some order and control.

Frank thought the whole thing was ridiculous, but was concerned about my job and my license. He urged me to get a written report from Dr. Bice sent to Betsy as quickly as possible, so that they might balance each other.

"I think I need to wait for an opinion of a psychiatrist, Frank. Betsy doesn't seem to value the opinion of Dr. Bice. Either she, or someone in the county, seems to think that a psychiatrist who's never met me can give a better evaluation of my mental status than a Ph.D. in psychology who's been working with me for months. Pretty ridiculous, but that's what I have to work with. I'll give Dr. Bice a call and see if he has the name of a psychiatrist he can recommend."

I lingered in the tension of that moment only briefly. The lack of control over my life had now invaded the last remnant of my old stability, my work, and all my rationalizing about things being in God's hands and for my own good felt like empty words.

But I still had my breath. At every moment, no matter how difficult, breath was there. Returning to it regularly, consciously, every day, had become an almost automatic response. I focused on my belly and took a conscious, deep, breath. And then another one, and another one. And a positive thought regarding my situation came to mind. Hadn't this situation given me the time I needed to rehab my leg with yoga? Wasn't I busy reading and enjoying this time off? Hadn't I started writing about these events? I'd always loved to write but had no time between work and the kids, and rarely had an idea worth writing about. God must have known I needed this time for something.

Before too long I was again comforted by the belief that everything would work out. I considered Dr.

Eugene's report to be simply a formality that would be resolved when I sought out a psychiatrist of my own choosing. That would be my next step. I did not think it would be difficult to find a holistically minded psychiatrist with whom I could work to resolve the misdiagnosis. With the shared the opinion of my psychologist, that I did not suffer from a major mental illness, it would be two against one and I'd be back to work.

Jade barged into my office where I was tapping away at my keyboard. "Mom, will you play a game with me? It's called *Spider's Thread*. It looks like the wall spider. It's on this board." He thrust his homemade game in front of me. "You'll be going from tree to tree and I'll be going from tower to tower."

"Wasn't Daddy going to play a game with you?" I asked him.

"He's playing with Iyra."

"Did you put away your clean clothes?"

"Yes," Jade answered impatiently.

Iyra stepped into my office. "Mom, do you want to try out the new shovel we bought you to garden with?"

"Not right now. I'm trying to write, and Jade wants me to play a game with him." I turned back to Jade. "O.K., I'll play one game." Jade played aggressively and defensively in just the right places. He is so sharp, and he loves to win. But it was time to get back to my writing.

Iyra came back.

"No, I do not want to climb up the ladder two stories to get onto our roof. I'm trying to write!" Frank stood behind her with imploring eyes.

Finally I gave in to their invitation for an opportunity to take in the view from the top of our house. I followed my family and walked through the office window to get out onto our backyard deck.

Windows as doors, I have no problem with this.

Chapter 8: Evaluation #1

We're thin people, just close the window behind you, please. But I am afraid of heights, and stepped tentatively rung by rung, gripping the sides of the aluminum extension ladder. I climbed like an old lady ascending stairs, dragging my weaker right leg behind my stronger left. It wasn't as weak as my heart. My hands gripped almost too tightly to keep going. Jade climbed on below me and began shaking the ladder.

"Cut it out!" I yelled to his grinning face. There is always the sensation of a vacuum cleaner sucking out my insides when I climb higher than about four feet.

I neared the top, and despite the urgings of my family, opted to absorb the sweeping view from the sure grip I had on the ladder. The view was an unobstructed one of the trees and valley a mile below. I faced west, and the air was clear and crisp. The frenzy of the busy city life was camouflaged by the density of trees. There are no tall skyscrapers in this direction, and the suburbs and shopping centers are somehow hidden from view. The coastal range of indigo hills rolled softly along the horizon.

Slowly I made my way back down the ladder. Wimpy leg, stronger leg, step, together. Step. Together. Hard to believe that only twenty years ago I rappelled down ninety foot mountain sides and jumped from an airplane with a parachute strapped onto my back.

I was scared then, too. For a while. Until I let go.

Chapter 9
The Reports

May 17.

    I allow myself to experience erroneous understanding in order to experience deeper understanding.

    Monday I would like to calmly walk into Betsy's office. I would like to be armed with my newest book by Dr. Gersten, *Are You Getting Enlightened or Loosing Your Mind?* and Dr. Dossey's book, *Healing Words: The Power of Words and the Practice of Medicine*, and perhaps even some flowers. Betsy works hard, and having given me the gist of the information ahead of time, I've been allowed to let my fury dissolve and to be considerate instead of pissed off.

    There is a way to flow through life without so much fighting.

    The Tao talks about the Way. It describes it

Chapter 9: The Reports

so clearly that I was captured by its purity and sincerity long before I was ever able to understand what it takes to live that way. The way. To be like a river, yielding, yet ever moving forward, carving canyons, moving mountains. Patiently.

A noble enough goal in life. God knows how far I am from being there most of the time.

In the height of my mystical experience everything was so clear, but clarity has become a little turbid now that I'm back to my usual self. Frank seems argumentative tonight. Should I yield? I speak up for myself, as kindly as I can.

When I speak my piece/peace, I begin to find it even in turmoil. If I stay quiet I can feel the turmoil build.

We can create only ourselves.

By our choices, we become who we desire to be.

I let the negativity wash by. I notice it. I notice my feelings, and for a change, I share what I feel.

A tree falls in a stream and clogs the flow. The water pauses for a while, understanding where it is, building from itself until, finally, it finds a pathway through, and onward. Pausing for obstruction, it is always itself, and there is always a path.

I hope to flow through my meeting tomorrow. I hope to be grateful for any further time off required of me. I can use it. There are never enough hours in a day, and I have dreams that are sprouting,

Ghostwoman

interests that are growing, myself to be exploring and becoming.

My friends are concerned for me. My job, my license. Somewhere inside, I must be a little frightened of these things, too. But there is a deeper calm that flows. The knowing that there is Divine purpose— to Everything.

The water flows with just enough turbulence to allow the river to know itself.

I met with Betsy in her downtown office. An uneasiness gripped me, but this was tempered by the parking space to which my thumbs led me. It was just across the street from the building and the meter still had time left, which was perfect, as I had very little change. Parking spaces seemed to be one of the last effective uses for the genius of my thumbs.

Eighth floor. "Excuse me, I have an appointment with Dr. Charleston."

Betsy walked out to greet me and we exchanged friendly hellos as she led me to her office, a fairly large space in the center of the floor.

"Here Betsy, I brought you a little present," I said, handing her a small blooming cactus. I wanted to do something to make the meeting a little more pleasant.

"That's really sweet of you," she said, taking the little plant from me. "But I don't think you're going to want to give me any gifts after all this."

"I can understand your position; you do what you have to do. I don't think I can understand this psychiatrist's perspective, however."

"Have a seat," Betsy said, pointing to a chair that was up against a wall." A woman from the benefits department will be joining us in a little while. She'll explain the leave you'll be on, and bring the paperwork

Chapter 9: The Reports

that you need to sign so you can get paid."

Scanning the office, my eyes fell upon one of Betsy's numerous books. *Healing Words.* "Have you read that book by Dr. Dossey?"

"No, someone gave it to me, but I haven't had the time to look at it."

"I'm just finishing it. Great book. Worth bringing on your next vacation." I sat down and looked at the book in my hands, which I'd brought along in case Betsy was running late, *Are You Getting Enlightened Or Losing Your Mind?* "I just picked up this one. It sort of jumped out at me. I like the title. The guy who wrote it is a psychiatrist."

"Looks interesting. I wish I had your time to read," she said.

Betsy pulled up a chair in front of me and proceeded to tell me about a chart review she'd done on all of my patients during the time period in question. I felt embarrassment for having been the cause of this extra burden. Small wonder she had no time to read books.

The benefits woman came in at some point and sat down to my left, listening quietly to our discussion, which unnerved me a bit. Betsy had uncovered no negative patient outcomes, but she found some errors in my charting, my more creative patient descriptions, and had an issue with my medical decisions on two accounts. I disagreed with her in both of these cases, related to the same drug, which supposedly differed from the general class of medications she was arguing about. I stood behind my choices of medications on these two complicated cases, and I even had a whole journal at home which I believed would support my drug choice.

"I'm not sure, but we're not here to argue about the drug. The reason for our meeting is the report I received from Dr. Eugene." Betsy handed me a five page copy of Dr. Eugene's evaluation. "I think you ought to read it."

"I'd like to take it home and read it if that's OK. Could you just summarize the points?"

"He believes you have bipolar disease and had a manic episode. He felt that you were still impaired during your evaluation. And he thinks you need to be on Lithium."

"That's a gross misdiagnosis!" I responded angrily, my eyebrows knitting together, the tension knotting up my shoulders and stomach. Then I remembered how common it was for manics to deny they have a problem and refuse treatment. It was considered to be a characteristic of the illness. "I don't have that illness." I said these words, realizing that they would float away and dissolve like a cloud. My credibility was gone.

Betsy was sitting across from me and talking without moving much at all. Only her head seemed to nod and bob for emphasis. "I respect your difference of opinion. However, if you want to keep your job, you need to be under a psychiatrist's care within thirty days."

"I'll be more than happy to see a psychiatrist, but *I* will choose which one."

"Of course," Betsy said, then added sincerely, "And I'm open to other opinions if you find a psychiatrist who disagrees with Dr. Eugene. In the meantime, I'm bound by law to report this to the Board."

Then we switched over to the details of how my benefits would cover me. First my sick leave would be used up, and then the disability for long-term illness would kick in.

"It's a three-month leave which can be extended if needed," Betsy added.

Three months? I thought to myself, feeling totally confused. Did she think I was that wacky? How could I seem so unstable to her and so normal to everyone else in my life?

Betsy walked me out to the waiting area and I turned to thank her for being open to a second opinion. We gave each other a restrained hug, then I turned and headed toward the elevator.

Chapter 9: The Reports

Breathe, Harriet, breathe. It's all for the best. Heart pounding, palms sweating, I stepped outside into the refreshing air. I felt like I'd just been released from some sort of prison.

Once home, I settled down with a cup of tea, and pulled out Dr. Eugene's report. All my meditation and breath work could not calm me. His words felt like an abominable distortion of my experience, like an old-growth forest turned into paper pulp. Exaggerated, focused on a pathological interpretation, he even seemed to invent things that I never stated. They were minor points perhaps, but points that helped to twist the interview so that I could more easily be stuffed categorically into a major psychiatric disorder.

K. Eugene M.D. PSYCHIATRIC P.C.

Harriet Cohen
May 7, 1998

. . . HISTORY AND MENTAL STATUS

In previous good health and normal occupational functioning, Dr. Cohen developed anxiety and preoccupation with marked ambivalence or indecision in the fall of 1997. These feelings focused on questions of home remodeling and/or purchase of a new home. Severe depression with symptoms developed in September, 1997, at the time of closing on a new house that her husband wanted but she no longer did. A freak accident in which she was struck by a car occurred on 10-3-97 and Dr. Cohen sustained leg fractures which required hospitalization and surgery. It is significant that her depression was so painful, she considered her physical injuries and recovery "nothing" in comparison. Significant depression continued for many weeks. Major depression then began to give way to fascination with the pursuit of enlightenment in spiritual healing, eastern or non-traditional views of health and illness, and a number of new-age authors. She attempted to limit herself to reading books by authors identifying themselves as M.D.'s.

Ghostwoman

Depression led her to seek help from clinical psychologist David T. Bice, Ph.D. According to Dr. Cohen, her psychologist encouraged and partially directed her reading in the new (to her) beliefs. It appears at least from her account that her psychologist may have conceptualized her depression as indicating a need for more spiritual or holistic viewpoint, or alternatively was supporting her own new interest in that direction. It is unclear from Dr. Cohen's statements what if any mental disorder was diagnosed at that point. She was also introduced to hypnosis and to the practice of observing her thumbs for spontaneous movements which would, she believed, provide her with answers and guidance. At some point prior to the onset of acute mania, she acquired a delusional belief that God was in this way communicating answers and practical directions to her, even as to her day-to-day activities. Personal decision making became unnecessary, replaced by following directives from somewhere, she knew not for sure where, yet she trusted the process blindly. Immediate give and take conversations with God, including questions and answers, were transpiring, she believed. She began to implement this practice in the conduct of her affairs, including for example on a shopping spree.

Sudden onset of acute mania occurred on March 29, 1998, during meditation immediately after a marital quarrel. Euphoria if not ecstasy accompanied a profound sense of oneness with all things. Extreme energy, marked increase in all passions (her term), joyful enthusiasm to communicate new insights to others (e.g., her patients), and a decreased need for sleep were all present. During this time her euphoria and newfound revelation spilled over into her contacts with patients, and this quickly came to the attention of colleagues and supervisors. Her conviction in her ability to communicate and to receive communications with God continued. The manic episode lasted ten days.

Now Dr. Cohen reports more normal mood and no recurrence of depression or mania. She continues to view all that has happened to her as part of a journey to enlightenment in some way. She has temporarily avoided meditation but values her talks with her psychologist, which she experiences as highly gratifying. She continues to esteem the practice of observing her thumbs, although at

Chapter 9: The Reports

times now is beginning to equate the term "God" with "intuition," in some way difficult for her to explain.

Family history of depression, bipolar illness, suicide, or alcohol abuse was denied. Past psychiatric treatment was denied. Ambivalence as to career and marriage were mentioned by her numerous times, and discussed at some length. No substance abuse history was uncovered nor suggested. Her physical health has seemingly been good.

Dr. Cohen's mental state currently is not euphoric nor agitated, it is mostly appropriate, and she is still loquacious but not densely pressured. Some flight of ideas remain at least intermittently. Dr. Cohen remains highly intellectualizing and rationalizing, yet coherent. She is aware now that her actions and words may not be received by others in the same way that she herself views them or intends them. Pressure to enlighten or educate others continues. This was evident even in our interviews. This further demonstrated a continuing grandiose and somewhat domineering mental position. It also demonstrated apparent unwarranted assumptions, disregard for potential negative consequences of her actions, and a seeming lack of awareness of other's wishes or reactions. She did request to be informed prior to my appraising the State Board of Medical Examiners about her condition, if such were necessary.

CONCLUSIONS

Based on my psychiatric assessment, my opinion is that Dr. Cohen has a Bipolar Disorder, type I, with onset probably in the summer of 1997. She first experienced a major depressive episode beginning late September, 1997, but probably was experiencing some prodromal symptoms weeks or months before that. Her major depression episode was followed by a true manic episode beginning rather suddenly on or about March 29 and lasting ten days.

Bipolar Disorder, type I, means there is a recurrent mood disorder with episodes both of mania and severe depression. It is my opinion that at least one of her symptoms was psychotic/grandiose, referring to her delusional belief regarding communications to her from God through the movements of her digits. Marked impairment in her occupational functioning was present during her manic episode.

As discussed in DSM-IV, a significant minority of persons with this disorder do show some residual impairment during intervals between episodes. Dr. Cohen does continue to show some residual impairments, which are most subtle but very much present. Hers are similar in quality if not in degree to her behaviors while in her previous manic state. I refer here chiefly to some pressure to evangelize, inappropriately and with some impairment of judgment, seemingly unconcerned with or minimally concerned with how this is being perceived by others. This is in spite of potential negative consequences to her. Another residual impairment is the persistence of her delusion noted above. A third is that she expressed looking forward to her employer/supervisor complying with her wishes that her supervisor and perhaps the whole clinic organization receive education and enlightenment in the new realm of spiritual healing and such that she has recently come to.

The prognosis in a Bipolar Disorder, type I, is described in DSM-IV, which I would add is consistent with our own psychiatric experience. The reality is that there is a substantial risk of recurrence of manic and depressive episodes. In light of all the above, it is my opinion that Dr. Cohen is in need of psychiatric treatment and help, and will probably remain so. As you know, it is most characteristic of Bipolar Disorder that the person so affected refuses or is simply unable to view himself or herself as ill or in need of treatment.

RECOMMENDATIONS:

1. My opinion is that Dr. Cohen is at present still impaired from her Bipolar Disorder. The degree of her obvious impairment may easily and rapidly change in either direction. It is my opinion that her condition has not yet improved or stabilized enough for her to return to work yet.

2. It is my opinion that one necessary condition for Dr. Cohen's successful return to her occupation will be ongoing psychiatric treatment. In Bipolar Disorder, type I, this

Chapter 9: The Reports

includes primarily medication, with lithium being the prototype. Verbal counseling will likely be of no help (at best) and potentially harmful, in the absence of appropriate necessary medication. This is not an arbitrary condition of employment, because even with treatment there will remain a risk of recurrent episodes, and the realistic goal of treatment is to reduce the risk, frequency, and intensity of the episodes. Without treatment it is likely that further episodes of mania and depression will occur—possibly suddenly, and more probably sooner than later.

3. Dr. Cohen should be advised to undergo a physical assessment to rule out possible organic conditions which can mimic a new bipolar condition (e.g., thyrotoxicosis, neurologic conditions, etc.) Onset at age 40 makes this even more necessary.

I trust this answers the questions you needed me to address. It is my hope that Dr. Cohen will fully recover and return to her regular occupation, which prognosis is well within the range of possibilities.

Respectfully submitted,
Gene K. Eugene III, M.D.
Diplomat
American Board of Psychiatry and Neurology, Inc.

I called Betsy after I finished reading the report and told her what I thought of it. "Could you do me a favor and refrain from sending it to the Board until I have a rebuttal written, and a second opinion from a psychiatrist of my own choosing?" I added.

"I think I can," she reassured me. "But I'll have to send some sort of a report to the Board in the interim."

5-20-98

It is a rather rainy day. Soft petals of water fall from the sky. From my house a sea of clouds covers the valley below, reaching far back to the horizon. It looks like the tide has come in.

The outcome of any situation creates new worlds of possibilities. We have the power to create "goodness" from any outcome. It is up to us to create it.

Mondeau plays with me. She interrupts me from my work. "I am a puppy! I am a puppy! Please play with me!!!" She has been so good today— snoozing, eating, hanging out, while I worked on the kitchen and my letters and packages, etc., and now I want to write.

"I am a puppy, I am a puppy!"

I choose to put my computer to sleep. She is a puppy, a magnificent and sensitive one. I willingly (sort of) give her a few minutes of my time. She is satisfied with so little.

We play catch with a ball, but she won't give it up. "I have your chewy bear that Grandma Eve crocheted for you!" She looks at me, at bear, and only then drops the ball to have a chance at the bear. Refusing to let go of the bear then... forgetting that it is a game— until she eyes the ball, and wants it, and drops the bear for a chance at the ball.

So we play.

And she teaches me about attachment, and the positive outcome of non-attachment— you get to keep playing the game!!! In the end, she gets both and goes to sleep.

Chapter 9: The Reports

Thursday, 5-21

A school book fair

—painting a good picture

—Lunch with Goretti. She gives my self-esteem a boost by telling me she wants a physician like me who integrates the whole person into the evaluation of illness and the creation of health.

—Then home. Running late en route to picking up Jade from school, I drove up my driveway to find a strange car parked in front of our garage, and two young women stepped out of it to talk to me. I have no idea how long they'd been waiting. They were dressed conservatively, one in a straight skirt, the other in slacks. They were from the Oregon Board of Medical Examiners and had two documents they wanted me to sign. I think I should probably have had a lawyer, as they are written in legalese. One looked reasonable to me, stating that I agree to not practice medicine until this whole mess gets resolved. Part of their document states:

"At the conclusion of the Board's investigation, Licensee's status will be reviewed in an *expeditious* manner to determine whether she may be safely returned to the practice of medicine. That review may take place by telephone conference call during a meeting of the Investigative Committee of the Board or during a regular quarterly meeting of the Board, but such review will not be unreasonably delayed."

I signed this document, but refused to sign the release of information for Dr. Eugene's report.

Thanks, but no thanks.

Ghostwoman

Two days later I received the following in the mail:

MULTNOMAH COUNTY OREGON
CONFIDENTIAL

May 18, 1998

Dear Harriet,

With this letter I would like to summarize the main points of our discussion today.
*   Dr. Eugene had completed an independent psychiatric examination of you to determine your fitness for duty. He is of the opinion than you are currently suffering from Bipolar Disorder, are currently impaired and cannot safely return to the practice of medicine at this time.
*   His opinion is supported by the findings of my investigation of multiple patient complaints and staff concerns regarding your practice and behavior during the first week in April. We have already discussed the results of that investigation, which are included in my memo to you of 4/10/98. His finding is further corroborated by results of an audit that I performed on all your patient visits which occurred during the first two weeks of April, up until the beginning of your leave of absence on April 20, 1998.
*   I cannot permit you to return to work until you have engaged in a treatment regimen for your Bipolar Disorder with a licensed, practicing, allopathic, psychiatrist. You can return to work when I have written assurances from your psychiatrist that you are no longer impaired by your Bipolar Disorder and that you are involved in ongoing psychiatric treatment and monitoring.
*   As of May 18, 1998, I have granted you a three month FMLA leave of absence. At the end of that three months we will evaluate your need for extension of the leave up to an additional three months.
*   Continuance of your leave and any extensions I grant you are contingent on your entering into psychiatric treatment and on regular progress reports from your psychiatrist.
*   My expectation is that you will enter into psychiatric treatment within the next 30 days.
*   You may seek a second psychiatric opinion and I will take those findings into consideration. The County is not

Chapter 9: The Reports

responsible for funding a second psychiatric evaluation.
*   I am obliged by law to report your condition to the Oregon State Board of Medical Examiners. I will proceed with that report following our conference today.

I understand that this is a very difficult period in your life. I am very concerned about your well-being and am anxious to do whatever I can to facilitate your early and safe return to medical practice. Please let me know what I can do to help.

Best Wishes,
Betsy Charleston, MD
Medical Director

5-23

The letter arrived from Betsy today, along with a copy of the letter she sent to the Board. Though I was expecting it, I didn't expect such a strong portrayal of myself as this profoundly manic woman. I find myself disheartened and want to write my rebuttal/clarification. NOW.

But there is a fight happening in the background between the kids over roller blades. And Iyra hasn't finished her chicken soup. And Jade. "You know how to cut up your own orange, you need to learn to be responsible for yourself," I tell him, though I know my desire for a healthy child filled with his daily allowance of vitamin C is more important to me than him cutting his own orange.

Iyra wants to go to OMSI, the Oregon Museum of Science and Industry. "It's the last day of the Omnimax Everest feature, Mom, we have to go!"

And I've spent all morning and half the afternoon at a swim meet for her and have grocery shopping

Ghostwoman

to do and dessert to make for our dinner tonight with friends. At least I don't have to cook the dinner. And I still have a cold and am a little tired and grumpy and hurt, and tired of people distorting a beautiful experience I had into a state of dysfunction and pathology. That is what makes me most tired.

    I need to meditate. After the laundry and the desserts are made.

CONFIDENTIAL   May 18, 1998
To: Board of Medical Examiners
Re: Harriet Cohen, MD

Dear Sirs:

I am the Medical Director for Multnomah County Health Department and in that capacity I serve as the clinical supervisor for Dr. Harriet Cohen. The County has employed Dr. Cohen to provide primary care to an adult, ambulatory population since 1985, I have been her supervisor since 1988. Dr. Cohen has been a good employee and is generally regarded by her peers to be an excellent clinician. She has a loyal following of patients.

It is therefore, with a great deal of regret that I report to you my belief that Dr. Cohen is currently impaired due to previously undiagnosed Bipolar Disorder and does not, at this time, possess the capacity to safely practice medicine.

To the best of my knowledge, Dr. Cohen was functioning normally until about April 1, 1998 at which time staff noted a personality change and what they considered inappropriate notes in the chart and difficulty getting appropriate answers from her in response to questions. Over the next few days clinic management received complaints from four different patients who had seen Dr. Cohen. Clinic management forwarded the complaints to me for investigation. Following chart audits, I met with Dr. Cohen on

Chapter 9: The Reports

April 8 at which time she related to me her own impression that she was experiencing symptoms of mania. I subsequently placed Dr. Cohen on administrative leave pending psychiatric evaluation. I also completed an audit of all patient visits beginning in mid-March and up until her last clinic day, April 13.

My audit revealed a change in her record keeping that became especially noticeable on April 1. I noted multiple documentation errors, a pattern of unusually brief histories, infrequent physical exams and an emphasis on spiritual counseling as a mainstay of therapy. There were also a number of inappropriate highly subjective comments in her notes. Although there were a couple of cases that suggested poor clinical judgment, my audits have not uncovered any untoward patient outcomes.

I engaged Dr. K. Eugene, a psychiatrist, to perform an independent psychiatric examination of Dr. Cohen. His opinion is that she has bipolar disorder with onset of depression in the summer or fall of 1997 and onset of acute mania on March 29 lasting about 10 days. He feels she has some residual impairment and is not now fit to return to work. Dr. Cohen does not endorse the diagnosis of bipolar disorder.

I have reported all of this to Dr. Cohen and have asked her to seek psychiatric care to which she has agreed. I have advised her that I cannot permit her to return to work until I have written assurances that she is engaged in a treatment regimen with a psychiatrist and that her condition has stabilized to the point where she can safely return to work.

Please call if you have questions or if I can assist in any way.
Respectfully submitted,
Betsy Charleston, MD
Medical Director

Chapter 10
Rolling up My Sleeves

I wrote my rebuttal over the next ten days.

May 26, 1998

Dear Dr. Charleston, and the Oregon Board of Medical Examiners,

    Thank you for giving me the opportunity to respond to Dr. Eugene's report about the extraordinary experience I recently had, his evaluation of me, and my own interpretation of my experience. Quite frankly, based upon his report, I'd have to agree with him that bipolar disease is a strong possibility for that patient. However, Dr. Eugene's report is very distorted from my perception of my experience, and my interpretation of it. He makes presumptions, uses erroneous adjectives in describing my experience, and relates details out of context. He also leaves out significant details that clarify distinctions between the state of consciousness I was in, and states of consciousness associated with mental illness, particularly mania and bipolar disease. Again, thank you for giving me the opportunity to clarify my experience, and my interpretation of my experience, rather than solely accepting Dr. Eugene's

Chapter 10: Rolling Up My Sleeves

interpretation of these things. As always, I will be entirely honest about this experience, including the more unusual details, in their entirety.

Regarding the onset of the severe depression I experienced this past fall, I feel that Dr. Eugene's report minimized the external events that occurred at that time in my life. This feels important for me to expound upon, as the details distinguish endogenous illness from grief and loss-related depression. Dr. Eugene's report limits the source of my anxiety, ambivalence, and depression to a matter of deciding whether to remodel our old house, or move to a new house. This was hardly the only significant event in my life at that time, and I shared more than this in my interview with Dr. Eugene. During the month of September, my grandfather-in-law, with whom we were very close, had a stroke and died. Additionally, I had a very sad personal loss which I alluded to, but chose not to disclose details with Dr. Eugene. I have discussed each with my therapist at length. Now add to that, four days after the death of our grandfather, and one day after the deeply sad decision I made regarding my personal life, a freak accident, which Dr. Eugene glosses over. I was hit by a car while buying bread in my neighborhood bakery. A car crashed through the storefront and squashed me between the car and the display case, breaking my leg rather badly. I bring this up because for me, it was the sort of event that forces one to start thinking a little deeper about life, and the meaning of life, and fate, and in whose hands our safety truly lies.

Dr. Eugene's next misunderstanding is still in the first paragraph, where he states that my depression "slowly gave way to fascination with the pursuit of enlightenment in spiritual healing...." and attempting to limit myself "by reading authors identifying themselves as M.D.'s." To clarify, my depression was quite severe for approximately 8 weeks, exacerbated, no doubt, by my limited mobility. During this time I was committed to helping myself to heal in any, and every way, I could. I considered taking Zoloft, got on a waiting list for a therapist, followed the advice of my orthopedist, took myself to an acupuncturist, and saw a homeopath. And, I started reading literature to help me make sense of the spiritual questions that arose from my accident.

Ghostwoman

The Authors "identifying themselves as M.D.'s," include the following: 1. David Simon, M.D., graduate of University of Chicago, trained in Internal Medicine and Neurology, past medical director for neurological services at Sharp Cabrillo Hospital, and chief of the medical staff. Currently medical director of the Chopra Center for Well Being in California, author of *The Wisdom of Healing*. 2. Brian L. Weiss M.D., graduate of Columbia University and Yale Medical School, and currently Chairman of Psychiatry at Mount Sinai Medical Center in Miami, Florida. He had published thirty-seven scientific papers and book chapters at the time he wrote the book *Many Lives, Many Masters*. 3. Deepak Chopra, M.D., a well-known writer, lecturer, and physician. 4. Caroline Myss, Ph.D., author of *Anatomy of the Spirit*. Though not an M.D., she has a Ph.D. in theology, and has worked closely with Norm Shealy. M.D., a neurosurgeon who has spent time in academics, private practice, and chronic pain management.

In Dr. Eugene's second paragraph, he makes reference to my "new beliefs." In fact, most of my "new beliefs" were not new; I simply had lost touch with them in my frantically busy life as mother, wife, and physician. The books I was reading in large part simply validated old beliefs and presented novel implications of these beliefs in the realm of healing. My psychologist helped me come to the self-realization of the parts of my life and self that I had been sorely neglecting, including my spiritual self. Early in the course of my visits, depression was diagnosed by Dr. Bice.

Months later, after my depression had significantly improved and I was no longer clinically depressed, I asked Dr. Bice if perhaps there was something in my past which was keeping me from fully resolving my depression, as I periodically still found myself unexplainably quite sad for a day or two. We agreed to try hypnosis. During a session Dr. Bice was able to 'hypnotize' (I think this word can have different meanings for different experiences) me, and I was aware of unconscious movement in my thumbs, identifying with "yes" and "no" answers. The movement was very subtle. (This technique of utilizing the movement of the thumbs is well known in psychiatric literature, and the official term for this phenomenon is *ideomotor movements*.) At the end of the session Dr. Bice explained to me that I might be able to achieve a state of self-

Chapter 10: Rolling Up My Sleeves

hypnosis, and allow my thumbs to give me answers from a subconscious level.

As to the "...delusional belief that God was in this way communicating answers and practical directions to her..." I would first like to clarify, as I did with Dr. Eugene, who and what was communicating with me. I explained, or rather tried to explain, that it was something other than my usual state of limited consciousness and voluntary movement: that I believed it was my subconscious, and superconscious, an intimate part of universal consciousness. The exact "what" was not important to me, but I acknowledged it was information that was beneficial to me in clarifying times of confusion. I have since been exposed to the term and the science, of *Kinesiology*.

"Kinesiology suggests that who we really are is a virtually free-flowing energy system and this energy has the answers to all of our questions about what is keeping us from creating our intentions and then what to do to create them. Kinesiology is a way of accessing your deepest wisdom through your body. The body gives yes and no answers to questions that we may not know the answers to consciously."[1]

As to my belief that God was involved with this, I will clarify what God means to me, as I did with Dr. Eugene. God is the Oneness of everything. The energy of the universe. The energy of all that exists and the potential energy from which all creation happens. This was most profoundly experienced by me in that state of unitive consciousness, and it has been the main concept of my Jewish background with which I have always found a deep personal truth. As an energy concept, Kinesiology allows everyone of us to personally experience "God."

Dr. Eugene's next misunderstanding is apparent when he states that I "...trusted the process blindly," which was not my experience at all. I was in fact fairly objective in

---

[1] This definition is contained in the introduction of a paper on "The Essence Process" by Dr. Andy Hahn, a Ph.D in clinical psychology, and a faculty member in the graduate counseling programs at Leslie College and Northeastern University.

Ghostwoman

evaluating the information that my thumbs gave me. When I made use of my thumbs as guidance in my everyday affairs, I did so with trust, but I also observed whether or not the answers and outcomes that I received would be ones that my conscious mind would find agreeable. Though this was not always the case, during the time that I was in my altered state, my thumbs led me to "correct" and favorable outcomes about 95% of the time. I considered that perhaps the other 5% of the time I was simply not privy to the full ramifications of an answer. I also realized that about 90% of the answers I received were yes answers. In short, I was assessing the value and validity of the information that I was receiving in an effort to better understand the usefulness of this newly discovered phenomenon.

I shared my "shopping spree" example with Dr. Eugene as a story that I thought would exemplify the positive nature of my outcomes, when I used the guidance of my thumbs. This was clearly not his interpretation, however, and his report leaves out details, which I shared with him, that differentiate the positive aspect of my thumb thing from the pathology and dysfunction associated with the state of mania. When I hear the words 'shopping spree' used in the same paragraph as "...prior to the onset of acute mania...," I envision outspending the bank and purchasing items hardly beneficial to the purchaser. In my case, at a time when I had thousands of dollars in my checking account, I spent the sum total of $387.00. I took my daughter shopping for some clothing items she needed, and ended up additionally purchasing very reasonable gifts for my family. I let my thumbs guide me, and they took me to a great parking space (important to me since my leg is still healing), to all of these items (except my daughter's things, which she enjoyed discovering for herself), and <u>one</u> store which had all of these items. Everyone loved their gifts except my son, who didn't like the feel of the sweater I picked up for him and couldn't care less about clothing. I picked up a dress for myself that I didn't bother to try on before purchasing, and my thumbs told me would fit. I have since tried it on and it fits perfectly.

Yes, I still am humored by the spontaneous movement of my thumbs. Although the percent of "true" answers is now far less than when I was in my altered state of

Chapter 10: Rolling Up My Sleeves

consciousness, they still find me great parking spaces, and when set before a myriad of choices I know nothing about, like what kind of shampoo to buy, or whether it is worthwhile to bring up an unusual suggestion at a meeting, they give me guidance.

The next clarification I would like to make is Dr. Eugene's judgment about my condition in the first line of his third paragraph of *my* history, where he states "Sudden onset of acute mania occurred on March 29, 1998, during meditation immediately after a marital quarrel." I would like to be clear that I did not then, nor do I now think I had a sudden onset of mania, but rather a profound spiritual experience totally compatible with similar experiences of other non-mentally ill people, that shared some characteristics common to mania. Although I'm unsure of the implications, my heightened energy state was not a sudden state, but one which grew slowly over the next couple of days and which lasted ten to fourteen days in total. There was a definite sense of an altered state of consciousness, and for two days my sleep requirements dropped to about four hours a night. The following night, however, while still in this altered state of consciousness, I slept peacefully for my full eight hours, and was in fact quite tired. My "shopping spree" occurred during this time, as well as my usual household responsibilities... in short, I did all of the usual sorts of things that always fill my days, and I did them well, and without incident, or concern by my friends or family. I also worked during this time, and there I experienced both complaints and praise from patients and staff.

At the top of page three, Dr. Eugene states I reported no "recurrence of depression or mania." I never said I was manic in the first place, and what I reported was that I was not depressed, nor had I been since resuming my more usual state of consciousness. I shared my view that I believed that life is a spiritual journey, but did not refer to 'enlightenment,' as it was not a term that I had used to describe my experience. Regarding my meditation practice, I had avoided meditation during my altered state, as I found my state a little unnerving and thought it would more likely settle down if I avoided meditation. At the time of my visit with Dr. Eugene, however, I had resumed my practice,

Ghostwoman

without problem or unusual incident. I did use the word "intuition" to try to explain my thumb phenomenon, as I'd hoped it would offer Dr. Eugene a non-rational word that might be more acceptable to him. I borrowed this analogy from an article I had recently read, written by a psychiatrist, about similar sorts of phenomena. I shared this article with Dr. Eugene.

 Dr. Eugene next refers to my ambivalence to my career and marriage. His statement leaves the reader with the impression that I was, or am ambivalent about these aspects of my life most of the time. In fact, I have always felt very blessed to have the job that I do, and have been fairly happily married about 75% of my marriage. Dr. Eugene neglected to ask my how my marriage was doing after my unitive experience and I would like to share that specifically, because here, too, my experience differs from the state of mania. It was through my experience that I was able to come to some understanding about several smoldering, and previously unresolved, issues in my marriage. I was on the verge of leaving my husband, and that is no longer the case.

 Regarding Dr. Eugene's last paragraph of my history, it is too bad that we don't have a tape recording of our conversation, because I take offense to most of it. Dr. Eugene suggests that my speech was somewhat pressured, and that some flight of ideas remained intermittently. We were trying to cover a lot of territory in an interview which Dr. Eugene said, at the onset, would take one hour thirty minutes, and which took over one hour forty-five minutes, at which time I let him know that my parking meter had expired, and that I had a carpool of children to pick up from school in fifteen minutes. We finished the interview the following week after another hour, as Dr. Eugene had more questions he wanted to ask and issues he wanted to clarify.

 I have always been aware that my experience could not be understood in the way I understand it except by one who has had such an experience, and so perhaps I do get a bit verbose in trying to share explanations, metaphors, examples, and books in order to try to be somewhat understood. I am curious about Dr. Eugene's perception that I demonstrated a somewhat domineering mental position. Perhaps I tried to

Chapter 10: Rolling Up My Sleeves

educate him about mystical experiences out of lack of knowledge whether Dr. Eugene was aware of such states. He made it clear at the onset of my interview that I could only answer his questions, not ask any of my own. And as to my disregard for potential negative consequences of my actions, I was, and am, well aware of the potential consequences of my actions. I have, however, learned to let go of the judgments that Dr. Eugene assigns to those outcomes, as I have learned that in the bigger picture of our life, what is initially perceived as negative or positive may quickly change in its ramifications. I trust in truth. I experienced what I experienced. And finally, yes, I would look forward to learning more about, and helping to implement and objectify spiritual strategies for healing with my patients, and with all patients. Larry Dossey M.D. and others have led the way in documenting the extraordinary payoff in terms of improved health when spiritual lessons are taken to heart.

Moving on to Dr. Eugene's conclusions, with which I wholeheartedly disagree, I would like to elaborate on my work experience (which Dr. Eugene notes as "marked impairment in my occupational functioning"), since this is where the question about my dysfunctional state originated.

While I was in the state of unitive consciousness, or *Samadhi*, prior to my heightened energy state, many things I had read about and heard about through the authors I have previously mentioned became acutely clear to me. Related to my work was the profound understanding that the physical world, including disease, is all a manifestation of spirit. I therefore hoped, and felt, that one could work with a patient from a spiritual perspective in addition to the physical and emotional perspectives more usual to my practice, to help them heal their illnesses. I <u>thought</u> I was approaching this concept gingerly, but it took a very unhappy patient to point out to me that I needed to back off on the direct relationship of illness to spirit and approach it in a much more subtle way. Having never experienced an altered state of consciousness before, I stumbled a bit in my approach to sharing this healing tool with my patients. No complaints from patients occurred after I remembered that I always needed to come from the reference frame of my patients' beliefs. I never withheld conventional therapy from patients, and always gave patients a full range of choices

Ghostwoman

regarding how they wanted to approach the treatment of their disease. I had a number of patients who truly felt better after our conversations, and others whom I was giving new ways of thinking about their lives in a psychospiritual way, which were well received. During this time, I was also able to assist in an office emergency. A colleague of mine saw one of my patients (a walk-in, as my schedule was full), and diagnosed an acute myocardial infarction. This was a more difficult patient of mine, and true to her nature of taking little care of herself, she was refusing to allow an ambulance to be called, or to consider going to the hospital. I went in and spent time with her, worked through her issues about going to the hospital and was able to get her consent for us to call an ambulance to take her to the hospital immediately. I personally retrieved and handed her the nitro and the aspirin.

Staff complaints and concerns were related to my exuberant mood and the odd spiritual issues that I was charting. In fact, I had made the purposeful decision, although with more than a little trepidation, to chart what was going on in my counseling to patients, and my impression of patients, so that if there were any positive or negative changes that resulted from my counseling, I would have documentation of what I did. Also, I was charting in a way that was creative and more fun than usual.

Dr. Charleston has subsequently performed an audit of my patient encounters during this time and encountered no bad outcomes. She felt that my medical decision-making was problematic in only two cases. As I discussed these cases with Dr. Charleston, I stand by my choice of medications prescribed, and at worst, think the specifics to be controversial. The first patient was a chronic pain patient, whose past stomach pains had responded to Zantac, and for whom we have never documented ulcer disease. The medication I chose was Relafen, which is the only non-steroidal anti-inflammatory medicine that bypasses the gastric prostaglandin pathway. Similarly, my other patient, an elderly gentleman with severe R.A., was given Relafen along with his low dose methotrexate for control of a recent flare in his disease.

Chapter 10: Rolling Up My Sleeves

Dr. Charleston did uncover some atypical sloppy charting during my altered state, along with "terrible handwriting" (though I would be curious whether it differs significantly from other busy days— my home journal entries during this time do not demonstrate a significant change in my handwriting), and some more creative descriptions of patients than is considered to be appropriate, objective medical terminology. I do not personally feel that these errors created any sort of a safety hazard for my patients, or were indicative of poor clinical judgment.

Spiritual experiences are common enough that we need to distinguish them from mental illness. Although sharing some similarities with certain states of mental illness, there are profound differences that allow them to be recognized for what they are. I am grateful for the courageous publications by psychiatrists that help to clarify both the frequency of such experiences, and their distinction from states of mental illness. However, as I desire to keep my job, I have agreed to follow through with an appointment with a psychiatrist of my choosing. As to the recommendation of lithium, unlike spiritual counseling it is a powerful toxin to the kidney, and I would personally consider it malpractice to recommend it to a patient who was happy and functioning normally without drugs, such as myself. I hope that the field of psychiatry, as an entity, will soon recognize that spiritual experiences are valid, and refrain from over diagnosing mental illness and recommending unnecessary and toxic treatments to patients.

I thank Dr. Eugene and Dr. Charleston for making me aware of how difficult it is to explain spiritual experiences to a western-oriented mind. I hope my written explanation and subsequent psychiatric evaluation help clarify my belief that I do not suffer from bipolar disease, and that it is safe for me to return to my outpatient practice of medicine. Though I do not think it necessary, should I ever be privileged to enter this altered state again, I would agree to letting my boss know immediately so that she could audit my charts, if she so desired, and ensure no undue lapses in documentation or patient care.

Sincerely,
Harriet Cohen, M.D.

Ghostwoman

I let Frank read my rebuttal. He thought I put in way too many details and suggested I refrain from sending it as it was. Though I could see where he was coming from, I felt too defensive to disregard any of it. I'd labored greatly over this response, addressing every minute detail that infuriated me. But I valued his opinion and decided to wait until it was reviewed by the psychiatrist that I would soon see. I realized sending my opinion alone would simply be the opinion of a "mad" woman, and might not even be read. It was lengthy, and I knew that a common feature in mania was prolific writing.

June 2

Yin-Yang, the center of my heart. The center of Love. The heart of God?

I have been balking at the diagnosis and label of having bipolar disease. Today, in yoga meditation, my humored mind drifted into a comparison between bipolar and yin-yang. Perhaps instead of fighting a bipolar label, I should be honored! But I know better. And the implied state of dysfunction and disease that accompanies this psychiatric diagnosis irritates me so, not to mention the loss of my credibility. It's hardly the same thing as the non-pathologic dance of duality that the yin-yang represents.

I finally received a return call this morning from Dr. Laural. She was recommended by the first psychiatrist I called, who was recommended by Dr. Bice. The first psychiatrist didn't want any patients for whom she had to write a report. Dr. Laural didn't have a problem with that, sounded very sweet, approachable, and caring over the phone,

Chapter 10: Rolling Up My Sleeves

considers herself to be personally a spiritual person. However, after hearing the brief version of my experience, she made it clear that she works within the standard framework of psychiatric diagnosis, and so would be compelled to either share Dr. Eugene's impression, or at the least, diagnose me as hypomanic.

Hypomanic. "Help me with something. Is hypomania necessarily a dysfunctional state? Aren't people in a hypomanic state often very productive, creative and happy? Why is this considered an illness?" I asked.

Dr. Laural stammered and agreed with my lack of understanding. And she encouraged me to try someone else. She said I needed an advocate for my perspective and recommended a Dr. Paltrow and gave me his number.

6 pm. My call returned from Dr. Paltrow. A high, New York sort of voice.

He asked intelligent questions and seemed none too put off by my dilemma. He also told me that he'd worked with the Board as a consultant on a case, and had been before the Board himself due to some of his nontraditional approaches. With his balanced experiences, he's probably well acquainted with their proceedings. I was relieved that he could fit me in before our trip to Florida in twelve days. Otherwise I'd be outside of those thirty days that Betsy has given me to connect with someone.

I am grateful. To Dr. Paltrow's open mind, To God, To my husband who finished up the dinner preparations while I talked with Dr. Paltrow on the phone, and to the beautiful blue evening sky and the 72-degree temperature outside.

We ate dinner outside and met our neighbors. I had to stand on my tip toes to peek over their high fence. They seem like a very sweet couple.

For the first time in days, I'm feeling my stormy sea beginning to calm down.

Prior to receiving the first name of a psychiatrist from my therapist, I called the Oregon Board of Medical Examiners to find out if they had any psychiatrists whose opinion they particularly valued. I wanted to be done with this ordeal as quickly as possible and sought to make sure that I connected with a physician whose evaluation would be held in high esteem. I was told that there were no particular psychiatrists that the Board could recommend. After I found the name of a physician, however, I could call them back and find out if the doctor I had chosen was in good standing with the Board.

I called them back after speaking with Dr. Paltrow, and was told that he would be fine. The Board had no issues with this doctor.

June 3rd, 1998

How quickly the sea can change. I am livid. I yell at the kids. They frolic outside in the sprinkler, cooling themselves off while I fume inside. Today is the day to go with the flow. What flow? The flow of an unfair world outside me? Or the flow of anger that boils within? I am volcanic, erupting threats of dire consequences to my children should they not cease their fighting. "I'm tired of being the referee

Chapter 10: Rolling Up My Sleeves

for your fights! If you can't solve this yourselves there'll be no more sprinklers for the rest of the summer!"

"Who's been messing around with the computer?!!? I can't find anything!!! Where's ClarisWorks??!!" I'm so cruel.

I called last week to clarify my timeframe with the Board. The main investigator, Marie, was still out on vacation, and I spoke with her assistant, Vivi. I let her know where I was in the process of connecting with lawyers and doctors— waiting. I asked about the timeframe and she assured me that nothing would be done until I initiated things by sending in a report. Marie had reassured me the day she appeared in my driveway that the Board wouldn't consider my case until all the pieces were together.

So, why at 4:45 do I discover a message on my voice mail that the Board is meeting? Tomorrow! And they will be reviewing Dr. Eugene's report! And I'd answered all my voice mails only two hours before!

One of the other messages was from Betsy letting me know they'd called her and wanted Dr. Eugene's report. Despite what I thought was an earlier reassurance otherwise, she gave it to them.

Then Iyra brought me the mail. There was the letter from the Board letting me know that they'd be meeting to discuss my case tomorrow. It was first sent to my old address, then found its way to this home.

How odd that the investigators who want me to

Ghostwoman

immediately sign a legal document that should have been reviewed by a lawyer, know where I live, but the person sending important pieces of mail doesn't.

I feel violated and betrayed. By the Board. By my boss. By the system. By my own naiveté. I have cooperated fully only to be treated as a nonentity. Perhaps this is why so many people I know do all that is within their power to avoid any psychiatric diagnoses. They know that a label will get you treated differently.

I tried to rationalize what was going on through the perspectives of my books and what I was feeling physically. Stomach churning, third chakra focus. Illnesses originating here were supposedly related to issues of self-esteem, sensitivity to criticism, fear of rejection, or issues of self-responsibility. That one fit too perfectly.

I tried reminding myself that there was a good reason for all of this somewhere, that in the big picture this all would make sense. But that didn't feel real to me at the time it was happening. My initial intrigue with the situation had all but vanished as I was swallowed up by feelings of helplessness in understanding what was going on or of having any ability to effect the outcome of my circumstance.

Marie called with a message that evening while I'd gone for a swim— no cause for alarm. Nothing was to be reviewed, except why I agreed to sign a paper allowing them to temporarily suspend my license.

So why were they so desperate about getting Eugene's report?

The most sustaining thing I did during this time was to begin to craft my story. There was something about getting my story out, writing about all of this that brought me peace. As I focused on the flow of words and the craft

Chapter 10: Rolling Up My Sleeves

of telling a tale, the grip of my situation would temporarily subside. It was not unlike the process of meditation where observing thoughts and feelings takes on greater importance than the thoughts or feelings themselves. Somehow, shifting the focus diffused the energy. Looking straight into the pain with a desire to describe it helped take some of the sting away.

Then there was the bulk of my life that still distracted me: the end of the year swim banquet for Iyra's swim team that I'd volunteered to coordinate, gardening, Shabbat School meetings, settling Jade down in the middle of the night after he awoke from a nightmare. Not to mention the more mundane activities of motherhood: the never ending shopping, cooking, cleaning, and paying the bills.

At least things with Frank had settled down.

June 8

Mondeau sits in the grass outside and watches the birds.

Spent my yoga time baking two pans of noodle Kugel for Jade's moving-up ceremony and celebration. The sweet scent of cinnamon!

Got the kids off to school this morning in a fury of blaming each other for being late, and so forth.

Left messages with Betsy, the swim camp, the art camp— actually got to talk to a real person. Talked with Greg about taking care of Mondeau while we're away in Florida, called PCUN, left a message with the social action committee.

Left a message with my lawyer. I don't understand why it's taken so long to get the cell phone records from the woman who hit me. Some

Ghostwoman

kind of a phone cord was found in the bakery after the accident. It had to come from somewhere. If she has nothing to hide, what's the problem? And I don't understand why her lawyer is allowed to look over all my medical records, including my visits to my therapist. Isn't this stuff supposed to be confidential?

Time for a quick bite of lunch, office work, a swim, Jade's ceremony, carpool, REI for sandals for the kids and bathing suits.

I guess I'll meditate while swimming, it's the best I can do today. Tonight, if I am not too tired, my painting assignment needs to happen for class, and my 2- to 4-page writing commitment. The laundry mountain needs attention before it begins to compost. And I am like the wind, trying to blow things right.

June 10th

Finally had my first appointment with my psychiatrist. What a refreshing visit compared to Dr. Eugene!

Dr. Paltrow has had experiences of his own, and with his patients that validated mine. He's read many of the books I have, and has been studying this field of knowledge for years. He talked about my thumb thing, which he considers to be a well-known hypnotherapeutic tool.

He said I had a problem with politics, not mental illness. Then he asked me if I knew Galileo's life story.

Chapter 10: Rolling Up My Sleeves

Galileo was given a wonderful telescope around 1600. With it, the heavens further opened up to his awareness. He was so excited that he wanted to share his gift with his country and his people. So, he contacted the Church and there was a big gathering about his gift, and everyone was thrilled with this telescope.

While heading home he pondered the long-held belief of the sun revolving around the earth and had an inspiration. The earth in fact revolves around the sun!!! He raced back and shared his new realization with those who previously were lauding him.

He was placed under house-arrest, and there he remained for the rest of his life.

The power of Fear, of threatening someone's belief system.

I'm worried about the old house, which needs attention. Frank's been mowing the lawn, but the weeds are all coming to life. After eight months, still owning it is wearing on me. I'd left it up to God's will, handed it over to the real estate agent who was selected by the three quarters I flipped in the air.

Just be patient.

Last month my thumbs suggested it would sell before the summer. Patience, AAck!!! I've nervously asked again and again. Are you sure???? By the end of May??? They twitched me a "yes." Well, May came and went, and here we are.

What to do, what to do...

Feel sad and burdened and cry. And start getting

Ghostwoman

a bug that grips my throat.

The fifth chakra is located in the throat. This location is about surrendering our own willpower to the will of God. That, and honest but compassionate expression. They are related, when I think about it.

I remember Chopra's teaching on how to get closer to God, to Love. He didn't teach the wiggling of one's thumbs, but the listening to one's own heart, learning to know one's true feelings. Perhaps that is why my thumbs aren't working so correctly anymore— it's time for me to stop depending on them for everything, and to resume getting to know my heart. Do feelings include feeling tired in the middle of the morning?

With a full day of chores before me and a western work ethic behind me, I went back to bed. Tears welled up as I lay there. This simple action of listening to my body's needs, and acknowledging them with acceptance rather than judgment, was so new to me, so honest.

I slept for over two hours! And when I awoke, I did not feel like a lazy bum, I had energy and enthusiasm for the day!

Thank you.

It is one thing to be unconsciously filled with so much love that one only has it to give, to see God and the miraculous in all things; it is another thing to return to a more usual state of mind, filled with insecurities, neediness, limitations, and bad moods.

Frank and I started having problems again when I started speaking my truth, asking for the things that I wanted, a little fairness between our egos. Could he please

Chapter 10: Rolling Up My Sleeves

wait thirty minutes to begin practicing the piano until I finished writing with my own music in the background? The piano is right on the other side of the wall where I'd been working, and the repetitive practicing was disturbing my train of thought. I was only asking for thirty minutes more. In a strange way, Frank's answer was not nearly so important as finding the courage to make my simple request. This was a good thing, too, as my request led to an argument, as if inspiring my budding courage to grow that much more.

This was another paradox: connecting to the interconnected web of all by appreciating the perspective of my own little ego. Defining who I was, not merely by the needs, wants and desires of others, but from a truthful place inside me. I was understanding ego not as a distorted part of self that considered itself greater than others, but as a unique facet of God that is AS important as others. It was up to me to chip away at the old patterns of thought and belief that kept this unique light from shining through me.

Then there was the issue of trying to understand the time and place for my ego, the time and place for egolessness, and the delicate balance between the two. Letting go had led to such a precious connection to God that I struggled with understanding how and when to let go. I had to learn not to let go of the things I could do, but to let go IN those things, and AFTER I had done what I could do. Letting go too early of things that I still had to complete only led to a very agitated state of mind.

A certified letter came in the mail. I thought it might be a bill, but it was formal notification from the Board that my license was suspended until my case was resolved. This was not unanticipated but still hit hard. What had seemed so clear to me was becoming clouded by the perceptions of others. It was as if I'd found an enormous diamond, knowing it could change my life and the lives of others for the better, then been told by a respected gemologist that all I'd found was a piece of petrified dung. Not only was the value of my discovery at stake, but my very ability to judge and perceive things was in question. And without that, I felt utterly useless.

Countering my despair with action, off I went to the library. I was looking for the psychiatric manual that defined my alleged condition, so that I would know precisely where to point out the error in my misdiagnosis. I was still of the misinformed belief that the *Diagnostic Statistic Manual* (DSM) was an objective text. The public library did not have a copy of the DSM, so I perused what they had that seemed potentially relevant to me. *Toxic Psychiatry,* by Peter Breggin. M.D. looked good, but was checked out. Another engaging title was available, *They Say You're Crazy; How the World's Most Powerful Psychiatrists Determine Who Is Normal,* by Paula Kaplan, Ph.D.

My family and I would be heading down to visit my parents in Florida in a few days. It would make good airplane reading.

Part II

"The mighty oak was once a little nut that held its ground."

Chapter 11
Validation

The kids grabbed the window seats, they always do. Frank sat next to Iyra, Jade and I sat in the row in front of them. Jade began pushing the buttons on his chair. "You can't lean back until after we take off," I reminded him. Backpacks were stuffed under seats, only briefly. Jade wanted his book, then just wanted to rummage through the pack. Decks of cards, new pads of drawing paper, books, snacks, drinks. Aha! Game Boy!

It was so much easier now that they were older. I settled down too, enjoying the quiet of the moment after the hurried morning of waking early and rushing to get to the airport on time.

I wondered when I'd have time to just sit and talk with Mom and Dad. I hadn't told them about the situation with my license and my work, hadn't wanted to worry them. I figured it'd be best to tell them in person, share things as they naturally came up. Perhaps the book I was bringing along would inspire a question or two, *They Say You're Crazy....* How could they not notice such a title?

Prior to opening Dr. Kaplan's book, I had never given much thought to how the psychiatric diagnostic manual was written. It had never dawned on me the power, the politics, the money issues, the sexual bias, or the degree of subjectivity that was involved in creating such a manifesto. When does depression become an illness, and when is deep sadness a normal human response? Under what conditions? If a child or parent dies, isn't it normal to be depressed? For how long? Why must *my* conditions for a "normal" sadness be the same as someone else's? And which label will mean my insurance will pay for it and which one means they won't?

I settled into my seat and began reading.

"Mom, would you play a game of cards with me?"

Mom and Dad were waiting for us at the airport. Jade and Iyra ran to them, and I could see everyone's eyes light up with joy and enormous smiles spread on all their faces. Arms opened wide, only to instantly wrap around each others' bodies in warm, tight hugs. Dad's cock-eyed teeth were so happy. He and Mom were tan and glowing. They never looked happier than in these moments in the airport when we got together after long months apart. We breathe full breaths, and the questions and the chattering are all so carefree and alive.

I had visited my parents the year before. It was my first visit without children, and part of my four-and-a-half-month, "heal thyself" sabbatical. I was exhausted from the previous twelve years of motherhood and doctoring. My weight had dropped and I couldn't seem to bring it up again, and my hands had a persistent low grade tremor.

My parent's home had been a place of peace and nurturing for me that year. The quiet was as delicious as Mom's cooking, and I basked in the simple joy of not having to tend to others for a while. My independent nature melted away, and I was too appreciative to even

Chapter 11: Validation

notice. Five days of being taken care of: of having love lavished on me, the care giver, the exhausted one. I began to put a little weight back on that visit.

But my parent's condo was not set up for children. Dining room chairs with wheels on them! Just don't move. You'll break the hand carved Japanese screen or chip the glass table. And be careful! Don't walk on the sliders for the Japanese screen doors! Dad's happy face quickly became pinched and twisted with concern as he chastised my absentminded, exuberant son, over and over again.

A glance in my direction. Did I imagine it? Wasn't it my responsibility to keep my children under control?

The kids didn't seem to mind the reprimands as much as I. But every rebuke out of my father's mouth hit me like a hammer. It was no longer just words, waves of sound that registered in my ears, but criticisms felt in my body as waves of energy crashing against me. Between my meditation and the mystical experience, I had developed, and continued to develop, a delicate sensitivity to my feelings. My emotions were alive, and like a foot that's been asleep and begins to wake up, the awakening was sometimes painful. The armor that I had erected over the first half of my life, to shield me from unpleasant states of being, had been removed; and I had not yet learned how to stay open and protected at the same time.

This did not make for an easy vacation, but a kaleidoscope of wonderful and strained visits with family and friends: my niece's birthday party, meeting a friend of my brother whose life had been saved by Frank years ago, when Frank stopped to help a stranger who'd been hit on his motorcycle and was bleeding to death (he'd never told me about that), outings to the beach, dinners with just me and my old best friends, the monkey and parrot jungles, laser tag and the like, was tempered by fragile emotions that stayed buried beneath pleasantness and only erupted during my meditation in cascades of tearful sobbing. All the issues that I thought I'd worked through came back to me in the stillness within my breath.

My sister-in-law, only a handful of years younger than myself, was pregnant with her third child. We could have had babies almost the same age. And another dear friend from high school who'd arranged to fly down and visit her own family at the same time so that we could see each other again, she, too, had just discovered that she was pregnant with a surprise third child. This saddened me, despite my best intentions for our world. But I shared this truth and sorrow with no one.

Then things got raw again between Frank and me.

We had left the strict order that my father required to preserve his home, not to mention his peace of mind, and were headed up north to see Frank's dad and his stepmother Thea. Driving away, I felt light and easy, like a bird released from a cage.

While Frank drove, I read to the kids from their chapter book, then gave my voice a break and read a bit to myself from Dr. Gersten's book. Dr. Gersten was the psychiatrist whose book helped differentiate spiritual experiences from mental illness. I was up to a chapter on visual paranormal experiences, which I found quite interesting, though I'd never experienced them myself, and I was inspired to read a couple passages to Frank. He disagreed with the distinction between angels and ghosts that Dr. Gersten was making, and made insulting remarks about my book. Before long we were arguing about the validity of Gersten's perspective. Next thing I knew, *I* was being insulted.

It was one more judgment and I'd had all the judgment I could take. Like a sea anemone being poked once too often, I closed up. I had nothing more to say until it came time for me to read Frank the directions to his dad's new house. This I did flatly, with few words. By the time we reached his father's home, I couldn't look at Frank.

I managed a strained smile for our hosts, who came

Chapter 11: Validation

out to welcome us warmly, then I said I'd be back to unpack the car in a few minutes.

"I need to stretch my legs for a bit."

Then I left them all visiting in the elegant new home while I walked and walked up and down the street and around the block. I could feel my eyeballs swelling, wiping the tears away before they burned visible tracks into my cheeks.

Frank had no hesitation finding fault with me and pointing it out, but it was rare for him to give me a compliment or say thank you for anything that I did. I had only recently become aware of this, and how painful it was to me, but I had yet to get up the courage to talk about it. Instead, I'd been deliberately trying not to criticize him, trying to make a conscious effort to give him the encouragement and gratitude that I so desperately longed for. If I was understanding Chopra correctly, the outside was a reflection of the inside, and I hoped I could clean up my outer life by simply becoming aware, then cleaning up my own behaviors. But it wasn't working.

Over the next three days I kept myself occupied with my meditation, my writing, the kids, talking with Dad and Thea, and calling old friends who lived nearby. It was easy enough to arrange myself so that I would not have to be near Frank. I even made sure we went to bed at different times.

I wrote volumes in my journal, trying to understand myself and get past my fear of speaking up. Who was he to be telling me what I think and feel?!?

Finally one morning while we were still in our room together I braced myself, holding back my fear so I could speak. I brought up what he's said back in the car, then told him his criticisms hurt and I'd appreciate it if he'd stop judging me.

"Well, I'm not going to keep it in. You want me to hold it in and get an ulcer?"

I didn't know what to say, and in my silence, he left

the room. Having only recently become honest enough to feel my feelings, I was still quite confused about them. I agreed with Frank that it was unhealthy to suppress our thoughts and feelings, yet his response made me feel worse! His lack of acknowledgment of my feelings, words of apology, or emotional support, further tore open the deep hole inside of me that was formed of feeling unloved and uncared about.

I could not put this into words to talk about it at the time. Instead, my pit simply filled with the desire to run away. I'd had enough of our relationship. And resolved to move back into the old house when we returned home.

That was when the offer came in for the house. A serious offer. Damn! Why then? My resolve had not fully crystallized just yet, and I was torn with the desire to get the old house sold.

It is interesting to me, how the Universe has always stepped in at the moment when my relationship with Frank was in the greatest trouble. The last time was back in the beach house, where again I was so determined to separate from him. Then came the breath that filled me with a love so whole and pure, that I needed nothing from anyone on this human plane. In that moment my feelings shifted completely, from wanting to desperately leave him, to wanting to be with Frank just so that I could love him.

That was not the first time, though. The first time happened before we were married. We were living on opposite sides of the coast in a long-distance relationship that was not working out, so we'd agreed to date other people. I'd met a beautiful man while lap swimming, and we made a date to have dinner. After talking for four hours like old friends, he drove me home and kissed me goodnight in the doorway of my apartment. It was 11:30 pm as I locked the door behind me. The phone rang; it was Frank. It was 2:30 in the morning his time, three thousand miles away in Miami. He'd had a dream that a prince was taking me away from him.

Chapter 11: Validation

6-20

No word about the house. And our counter-offer expires today. I have been holding back tears all visit. I ask myself if I should move back into the house. My right thumb twitches forcefully, NO.

Maybe? I plead.

NO.

Tears well up. Nowhere to go. I wear a little smile and wonder why I have such low energy (except when I visit with my old friends).

Why? Why? Why?
Why are we so apart, when we
were so close only yesterday.
Or was it last month, or the month before?
But we drifted
despite my best attempts to remember how
to stay united
is so difficult.
When you go on forever, there is no running away.
No stepping out.
There is so much to learn
And it is so impossible to learn alone.
And to know the truth
Is so miraculous!
and so difficult to understand and become
Unconditional Love.
Are we moving towards the light? Yes.
Do I have to keep touching the darkness? Yes.

I am tired of my sadness. They are all so happy....

watching Bugs Bunny.

Ghostwoman

They laugh.
I smile my Mona Lisa smile.

6-21

I don't want to hear anymore "You should have's..."!!!!!!!!!!!!

6-22

We drove back to my parents home yesterday. Last night we lay in bed and talked about my coldness. Frank was the one who started the conversation for a change. His caring enough to bring it up allowed me to share what I felt, and have been keeping inside of me.

Again, I asked him to join me in marriage counseling.

He shared why he didn't want to go— he'd be too inhibited. Yet, he wanted to know what my therapist thought.

I tried to explain that therapy is not about what the therapist thinks. It's about helping me to think and feel things that I had not had the understanding, or courage to feel and think about on my own. Dr. Bice asked me questions that allowed me to see my blind spots about my feelings. He helped me validate myself with his supportive, nonjudgmental way of listening.

Frank was still hesitant about opening up to a stranger, but not flat out refusing. I suggested that in the meantime, we consciously say something positive to the other person before disagreeing, or

Chapter 11: Validation

finding fault. He agreed to this.

We also agreed not to criticize the other person when we disagree with them.

I didn't mind my opinions being challenged, in fact, in moderation that could be stimulating, like a game of chess. What I could no longer stomach were my feelings being challenged. That felt like a direct insult to my truth.

Frank also agreed to apologize when I let him know that he'd hurt me. He felt that by saying "I didn't mean to hurt you," he was saying the same thing. It doesn't mean the same thing to me. We can feel sorry for something we meant to do, or not sorry for something we didn't mean to do.

He began to stroke my arm very gently. I traced little circles lightly on his chest and belly. Slowly we made love.

I dreamed that night about not liking our new house again. I dreamed about a house with a view of a snow-covered hill with palm trees growing on it.

It's morning. Frank tells me the best way to hang towels to dry, folded over so that there are only two layers of cloth. I tell him my way, carefully scrunched so that there is only one layer of undulating fabric. He tells me that I was hanging it <u>wrong</u> at Dad and Thea's house and that it annoyed him.

What happened to that agreement we made last night? I meditate again through tears, wondering if we'll ever get anywhere, if we'll ever get out of this ditch we seem to be stuck in.

I never did get the opportunity during the vacation to tell my parents what was going. Neither they, nor Frank's dad, nor Thea, asked about either Paula Kaplan's book or my work, and I didn't initiate that conversation. I didn't want to have to explain and justify myself. I saved those conversations for my visits with my friends. In their presence I could breathe fully and be myself. Sharing my extraordinary experience was a blessing to wonder about together, not an opportunity to label and gawk at as some abnormality or state of disease.

Yet, one of my oldest and dearest friends who was a psychologist, confided with me that she considered the diagnosis of mania. And though I appreciated her honesty with me, I felt her labeling create an invisible barrier between us.

* * * * *

Two days after returning home I returned to Dr. Paltrow's office for my next appointment. He focused on pulling together a complete picture that would, hopefully, satisfy the concerns of the Board. Having had dealings with them himself for using unconventional approaches to help patients, he knew that I was up against a difficult audience. To support his opinion that I didn't suffer from a major mental illness, he even suggested that I take a number of standard psychological tests to help objectify his position.

The three separate tests took hours to complete. There were sixty-four unfinished sentences, and over five-hundred true-false questions I thought had a profoundly sexist perspective. There were questions about hunting, but nothing about volunteering in schools, nurturing behaviors, or about spiritual values. The only part that was any fun was the unfinished questions which allowed a bit of creativity. A few of my favorites:

34. My greatest weakness is--- my greatest strength, depending on the circumstance.

Chapter 11: Validation

    35. My secret ambition in life--- is to create beautiful and interesting stuff, be happy, and help heal the world.
    40. I wish I could lose the fear of--- living, all the time. It is mostly gone, but not quite.
    41. The people I like best are--- spiritually aware and inspired.
    42. If I were very young again--- I would probably have to relive the painful experiences I've already worked through.
    55. My fears sometimes force me to--- not say what's on my mind.
    63. I like my mother but--- she still likes to tell me what to do.
    64. The worst thing that I ever did--- must have had some purpose...

    These tests would not be covered by my insurance, which was rapidly reaching its mental health limitation. And so over $600 later, we were armed with standardized evidence (God only knows how they standardize such subjectivity) that I,
    "...did not suffer from a medically significant emotional disorder..."
and with an MMPI that claimed to demonstrate,
    "...a valid profile but might have attempted to present an unrealistically favorable picture of her personal virtue and moral values; a rather naïve or unsophisticated self-view; the profile was within the normal range suggesting that she viewed her present adjustment as adequate; no clinical diagnosis was provided; one subscale elevation was that of inhibition of aggression."

    Or in my words: not crazy but with high moral values and a bit naïve and unable to feel and express anger (though I was beginning to learn).
    I could live with that. I saw some truth in this characterization of myself and was impressed, particularly since it had come out of such male-oriented questions.

The exam reminded me of the written Torah. It also had the capacity to reveal beautiful truths that sprouted from a male-oriented, often patronizing document. My precious, sacred text included the *Shema*, which beseeched the Jewish people to Listen! Listen for the Oneness of God! Love the Oneness with all your heart, with all your soul, and with all your might! Love your neighbor as yourself!

But such jewels, and more, were surrounded by a need to command the people to listen, with threats of dire consequences if we fell short. Such language kept me alienated, but I was softening to a presumption that this was the only language that the majority of the people could understand, back when the words were written.

On the floor of our bedroom, across from the foot of our bed, sat two old, round pillows. Sandwiched between Mondeau's big pillow bed and Frank's dresser was the only place in our small room where they would fit. Since my cast had come off, I'd been sitting on them for my meditation.

I developed my own little ritual of wrapping myself in an old, soft, cotton, Mexican blanket that had been a gift from my parents. I'd begun this during the cold winter months, and meditation never quite felt the same without it, even on hot summer nights. I'd sit on my pillows, facing east, close my eyes, and do some sort of a breathing exercise that shifted and changed over time, as I played with new techniques I would come across in my reading. Then I would drift in silence into pure observation of my breath, ten to thirty minutes. I'd feel it begin in the belly, feel the cooler air coming in through my nose, then watch all the physical and emotional sensations as the breath filled me, paused, then slowly emptied, paused, and began to fill again.

Some days I added a mantra. *Yod. Hey. Vav. Hey.* In. Out. In. Out... Breathing. Letting my thoughts blow away, trying to expect nothing.

Chapter 11: Validation

But a little disappointed when nothing came.

Why couldn't I return? I missed those days where fear melted into faith. I wanted to feel Unconditional Love again. What was I doing so differently now?

Back to Dr. Bice.

Back to Dr. Paltrow. He sat at his desk. I faced him in my chair. He had put together his report about me and asked me to go over it to make sure that he'd captured the events correctly. I stiffened as I realized he'd included my abortion. I could feel my face grow hot and uncomfortable, looked up at him and said, "I understand that you need to know about my abortion, to put it all in perspective, but I don't think the Board needs to know about that."

Dr. Paltrow sat forward in his chair and spoke slowly and clearly, "It's been my experience that when we try to avoid, or cover things up, that's when they're most likely to come flying back at us. Those parts about ourselves that we feel the need to conceal often become an unintended focus in our lives and in our psyches. Think about it. I don't think the Board is interested one way or the other in the abortion, but I do think it would help them to get the whole picture."

7-21

It took a couple days, but gradually my mood has lifted. Down a few days, up a few, here a day or two, gone again.

Whether it is the tears that Dr. Bice helps me shed in our sessions, or the visit with Cindy, or the stars, I don't know. But I know that I awoke today feeling happy!

I even had to miss yoga because of a flat tire and didn't get all wigged out. In such a lovely mood, I mostly felt grateful that I was allowed my flat in the comfort of my own garage and in the cool hours of the morning. It was only the second time I have ever had a flat tire, and I felt so proud of myself for changing it.

Gardening instead of yoga— I pulled up the spent and fallen snow peas. Then off to learn energization exercises at the Ananda church. From there to Dr. Paltrow, then the tire shop, where they fixed it for free!

Reading. An easy dinner. Writing. The day is 90 degrees and sunny. The house is warm.

And it is lovely.

What do these moods mean? Do I need to just accept the down times, or should I be somehow working through them? Trying to know their origins? Or both? The day has its night. The warm has its cool. Maybe I just need to find things to appreciate and value about the shadows. Take the time to allow the feelings of grief and sadness to move through me. Wholeness includes all the opposites.

In my subsequent and ongoing study of holistic medicine, I found repeated evidence and support for this understanding of wholeness. Chinese medicine includes a model of **all** the emotions as a circular path, where emotions are ever-changing. Joy evolving into sympathy, evolving into anxiety and sorrow, into fear, into anger, which revolves back into joy.

This capacity is underscored in *Remarkable Recovery*, by Hirshberg and Barasch—a beautifully written and scholarly collection of stories about very diverse people who experienced complete recoveries from terminal illnesses. A search for common features amongst these patients found the capacity to experience a full range of emotions nestled squarely in the beliefs and authenticity of the individuals.

Al Sieberts uncovered a similar capacity in his study of the personality traits of survivors of war. They are both serious **and** playful, logical **and** intuitive, hardworking **and** lazy, shy **and** aggressive, and so forth. It was surmised that this gave the survivors a wider array of resources to draw upon. The key to their survival, and to health, seemed to be an awareness and management of these various states of mind, not an attempt to limit the emotions to only the positive ones.

The old house sold in mid-July to a woman who loved it and had plans to turn it into a Wholeness Center. A Wholeness Center— in my old house! I could not have been happier, wanting the house to sell to someone who appreciated it as much as I.

Here I'd gotten myself into a mess through my use of hypnotherapy, my desire for wholeness, and my spiritual connection, and the old house was selling to a sympathetic reflection of all these things!

The buyer was a hypnotherapist who was working with another woman, a spiritual healer who did energy work. I felt validated by this uncanny connection, and the friendship that would grow supported me through my ordeal with the Board.

Weekly visits with Dr. Paltrow continued. It was a tedious task to have to review all the same details one more time, but Dr. Paltrow wanted the report to reveal my life in an unbiased and thorough manner. I'd given him the response I'd written, but like Frank, he advised me not to send it, to let his report speak for the two of us.

One reassurance that Dr. Paltrow was able to give me was in regard to my thumb thing. He'd done quite a bit of work with hypnotherapy over the years, and was quite familiar with the technique. He recommended a book on hypnotherapy by Dr. David Cheek, a gynecologist.

"What about hypnotic regressions?" I asked one day when we had a little leftover time. "Have you done much work with that?"

"I have. It doesn't work for everyone, but a number of my patients have had amazing healing through the use of that kind of therapy. One particularly memorable patient was a woman I saw in 1977, who was dying of an autoimmune disease, though her symptoms were controlled by prednisone. At age twenty-one she was given between six months and five years, to live. The circulation in her extremities was sort of shrinking, closing up. And this process was moving up through her body, from her hands and feet towards her torso. It was beginning to affect her internal organs as well. Not surprisingly," he continued, "the woman was depressed. Her physician referred her to me. I told him I would treat her depression by focusing on hypnotherapy with the patient."

Dr. Paltrow sort of rolled his eyes. "I don't think he was too thrilled to hear that, but he just said, 'Whatever.'"

He continued. "The woman was easy to work with and I was able to take her back to many previous lifetimes. Two in particular seemed related to her current medical condition. In one lifetime she was an Inuit woman, forced to flee from a hostile tribe that was approaching. She and the other women of her tribe retreated with the children to the sea in their kayaks. But the water was too rough and the boats overturned. The patient described the sensation of dying in the icy water, as the cold systematically numbed her hands and feet, moving proximally up through her body until she drowned.

"In another lifetime, this patient recounted another unpleasant death in which she dehydrated while in a desert. The symptoms had a profound similarity, numbness spreading from her periphery, proximally, until once again she was consumed.

Chapter 11: Validation

"After working through these past life traumatic deaths, along with gradual decrease in medication, the patient no longer suffered from the autoimmune disease. She and I both thought that the hypnotherapy contributed to her healing. In all likelihood, it was the combination of the medication and the psychotherapy that led to the resolution of her condition."

I was transfixed by Dr. Paltrow's account. I had read of psychological healing through regression therapy, but this was my first account of the strong connection between our transpersonal history and physical disease. It was one more piece of the mindbody puzzle that continued to fascinate me, and which I continued to avidly study during my forced leave of absence from work.

7-23

Dinner is done. The house is an ideal temperature. The sun is still out. The air, cooling off.

I have crawled inside my shyness again. How glorious it felt to not be shy for a little while. Shyness is fear.

Deer are shy... and other forest animals. Delicate. Wary of being eaten.

Otters aren't shy. Boisterous, bold and bubbly. Get too close and watch out! They know how to take care of themselves. They also know how to let you know so that no one has to be hurt. Hisssssss!!!!

I observe myself. If anyone asked me what I did these months off work, I would say that I observed.

This is quiet time. Though often too busy to fit in a yoga class, or writing. There are finally

Ghostwoman

pauses in my life. Pauses that sometimes drift away with a book in my hands, learning about things that have some meaning for me.

It was watercolor class today and my day to bring the goodies. I brought the banana bread I baked last night. I stayed up late baking and painting.

The first person to take a slice took two bites, then set it down and popped a piece of candy into her mouth. This is the dilemma one always faces when we create from ourselves: we risk rejection. Surely unfinished donuts would not have left such a feeling as the bread I chose to share with my classmates.

How pleasant when the rest of the class enjoyed the bread. It disappeared quickly. All that was left were requests for the recipe.

The music I brought along was also enjoyed. Linda even wrote down the names of both of the tapes. It feels so good to share a little taste of happiness. And so wonderful to be appreciated!

Why does it feel so good to be validated? Perhaps the answer is the same as the reason plants need water to grow.

Why? Because.

Chapter 12

Diagnosis #2

July 29, 1998.

$6.00 for 1 hour 15 minutes of parking!

What a slick law office Thomas McDermott has. A view of the surrounding city and hills from their 34th-story aerie. Marble furniture, expensive everything. I asked if they validate parking. Sure, but it just gets added to my bill. Gee thanks.

I like McDermott. He's a cute man with so much exuberance! A human version of an elf in a pin-stripped suit. Talks fast but seems to know what he's talking about and strikes me as having a lot of integrity.

I took up an hour of his time while he reviewed the documents I'd accumulated so far. He read the Board's order, Betsy's notes to the Board and to me. He read Eugene's report. He read my response. And echoed everyone's opinion that it is better left unread. "Give as little information as possible. Don't expose yourself."

No one has anything positive to say about my masterpiece. Ten days of work, carefully dissecting Eugene's despicable evaluation and setting my side of the story straight. I guess it still looks crooked to most people.

There's a new song on the radio that's often on while I drive from this place to that, "...All I need is a good defense, 'cause I'm feeling like a criminal....." I sing along with the chorus while I drive. It's better than the shower. With the windows rolled up I can sing it LOUD!!! It gives me energy and makes me laugh.

At my first visit, Thomas emphasized the tremendous amount of authority that the Board wielded. They were protected by various ambiguous ordinances and therefore enjoyed almost unilateral power in their governance. There were no hard-and-fast rules for how quickly they needed to resolve their concerns about physicians, and it had been Thomas' experience that unless physicians did just what the Board asked, they'd drag out the process and be particularly heavy-handed with their resolution orders. I wanted to return to work as quickly as possible and agreed to follow Thomas' advice.

Monday night, 8-3

I am filled with tears. I walked out of the room while talking to Frank because I didn't want him to see me like this again. Dr. Bice seems to have me ripping open Pandora's box.

It is so odd, I was feeling so together while

Chapter 12: Diagnosis #2

talking to him today, the visit went calmly enough. He suggested I come back in one week. I balked. Did I need weekly visits? I was feeling so good!

Now I can't stop crying again. Why? It started because I hurt. Physically. My fibromyalgia is back. I'm tired of hurting. Tired of being tired and having no inspiration, no desire, just being tired so much of the time. What did I do? Not much. A little this, a little that... finished getting the pictures ready to copy. Finished letters. Watered a little. Yoga. Not much.

I miss working.

I don't like feeling sorry for myself. So many people have so much less than I do. Less money, less love, more pain, more problems. My desires and inspiration fade into my fatigue or my pain or my fears of not doing a thing well enough.

I read all my books and I know them to be true- the importance of taking control of one's attitude towards life. Still, I can't seem to unlock myself from my fears and fatigue. How do I free myself? All I can do is read. This is all I know how to do. And meditate on my breath.

I wonder where I'll go nowhere today.

8-5

What a difference a day makes. Energy is back, a nice walk, a chance meeting and delightful conversation with an acquaintance along the way. Then my apt. with Dr. Paltrow, stopping on my way home for some fun little shopping in the village.

> Home, where Mondeau and her ball remind me once again about letting go. Catch is still her favorite game, but she returns with the ball only to completely resist giving it to me so that I might throw it to her again.
> Mondeau, if you don't let go, you can't keep playing!

Dr. Paltrow finished his evaluation of me and asked if I was I comfortable with his description of my experiences? Did I think it needed any clarifications or corrections? I did not have much to change, finding his report to be a fairly accurate retelling of my account, with only a few minor corrections. The only problem that I had with his evaluation was at the end where he gave me a diagnosis. He explained to me that he needed to give my experience some kind of a label which would be acceptable to the Board, something that could be found in the psychiatric diagnostic manual. He was confident that the diagnosis he chose and applied to my circumstances would be acceptable, and would not be likely to cause further problems for me, personally or professionally.

AXIS I: 309.9 Adjustment Disorder, unspecified. This subtype should be used for maladaptive reactions to psycho-social stressors that are not classifiable as one of the specific subtypes of Adjustment Disorder. The essential feature of an adjustment disorder is the development of clinically significant emotional or behavioral symptoms and response to an identifiable psycho-social stressor or stressors.
  The differential diagnosis includes Major Depressive Episode. For part "A" five of nine symptoms had to be present— she had four: 1. depressed mood, 2. markedly diminished interest, 3. fatigue or loss of energy, 4. feelings of worthlessness or excessive or inappropriate guilt. She did not meet "B," the criterion for a mixed episode. She did meet "C," that the symptoms caused clinically significant distress or impairment in social or occupational functioning.

Chapter 12: Diagnosis #2

As for "D," the symptoms were due in part to a medical condition— fractured bones of her right leg. As for "E," the symptoms were better accounted for Bereavements.
    She did not meet the criterion for a Manic Episode. The period lasted 10-14 days. She did meet "A," that being a distinct period of persistently elevated mood (spirituality). Regarding "B," during the period of mood disturbance, she met none of the following seven symptom possibilities. She did not have an inflated self-esteem or grandiosity; for two days she needed 4 hours of sleep and the days thereafter eight; she was not more talkative than usual nor did she have the pressure to keep talking; she did not experience flight of ideas; she was not distractible; there was no increase in goal-directed activity or psychomotor agitation; and no excessive involvement in pleasurable activities with a high potential for painful consequences—the buying of gifts came to approximately $387.00 and the purchases were realistic. For "C" the symptoms did not meet the criteria for a Mixed Episode. For "D" the mood disturbance did not cause marked impairment but rather a slight impairment in occupational functioning. And regarding her relationship with her spouse there was an increased openness— benefiting them both. For "E" the symptoms were not due to the direct physiologic effects of a substance or general medical condition.

AXIS II: No diagnosis

AXIS III: Post motor vehicle-pedestrian trauma, sustaining fractures of the two long bones in the right leg along with soft tissue injury. Pain occurs when carrying perhaps more than 10 pounds, and with long-term walking. There is absence of the majority of her recreational pursuits because of the musculoskeletal pain.

AXIS IV: Other psycho-social and environmental problems: the motor vehicle-pedestrian accident contributed to the kindling of the profound spiritual experience. Dr. Cohen had time to read to excess of the subject. She appreciated that it could have been a fatal accident, or could have caused more trauma and residual than she currently has. Dr. Cohen appreciated that the accident contributed to her concerns about safety anywhere— how can a pedestrian in a store be struck by a car? Thus the spirituality and concerns about the meaning of life for self and others.

AXIS V: Global assessment functioning: fifty percent serious impairment in occupational functioning because Dr. Cohen's license to practice medicine has been suspended.

FORMULATION:

Dr. Cohen, at the time of this writing, continues to experience emotions, physical pain, and limitations from the accident of October 3rd, 1997. Dr. Cohen continues to process all the pieces contributing to the kindling of the spiritual experience. Dr. Cohen did not suffer a Major Depressive Disorder or a Manic Episode as part of a Bipolar Disorder. She did suffer an Adjustment Disorder, unspecified. I believe she is competent to return to work for Multnomah County Health Department. I believe continued therapy through her psychologist, Dr. Bice, would be in order. In my opinion she does not need to be on any psychotropic medication at this time.

The prognosis is good. She has learned that moderation and limitations are necessary in her social, occupational, and spiritual pursuits.

Sincerely Yours,
Kenneth Paltrow, M.D.

    Overall, I appreciated Dr. Paltrow's evaluation and conclusion greatly. But I balked at his last line. Moderation and limitations may be necessary for certain outcomes, but alternative outcomes may in fact be preferable in the long run. Besides, one individual's excess is another's moderation. We are only as limited as we choose to be.

    But this was the final report, which was sent to both of my attorneys, as well as my boss. It was reviewed by Thomas McDermott, and forwarded to the Oregon Board of Medical Examiners.

Chapter 12: Diagnosis #2

August 7, 1998

HAND DELIVERED

Marie Wong
Board of Medical Examiners
620 Crown Plaza
1500 SW First Avenue
Portland, OR 97201-5826

        Re: Harriet Cohen, M.D.
        Our File No. 81983-0001

Dear Ms. Wong,

    This will follow up our telephone conversation of Friday morning, August 7, 1998. Enclosed please find Dr. Paltrow's August 5, 1998, letter to me regarding his treatment and evaluation of Dr. Cohen. Significantly, Dr. Paltrow concludes that Dr. Cohen did not suffer a Major Depressive Disorder or a Manic Episode as part of a bipolar disorder and that she is competent to return to the practice of medicine with Multnomah County Health Department.

    You indicated that before Dr. Cohen's license could be reinstated, it would be necessary for her to be interviewed by the Board's Investigative Committee and that the next opening would not be until Thursday, September 24, 1998. The Board has also requested a signed release from Dr. Cohen so that the Board can obtain all records regarding mental health services that may be relevant. It has also been requested that Dr. Cohen write a letter to the Board confirming her desire to return to the practice of medicine and stating her belief that she is mentally competent to do so. You also asked that the letter confirm that she has a treatment plan in place or an explanation of why she does not feel such a plan is necessary.

                            Yours very truly,
                            Thomas E. McDermott

cc: Harriet Cohen, M.D.
    Kenneth Guy Paltrow, M.D., P.C.

    Then Thomas sent me a letter, outlining the next steps that I needed to take so that I could be interviewed

Ghostwoman

by the Investigative Committee at their next meeting, Sept. 24th. Even so, Ms. Wong indicated to him that mid-October would probably be the earliest that I would be able to return to my medical practice because the Investigative Committee would have to make a recommendation to the Board following my interview. Then the Board would have to vote to reinstate me.

One more month, when every week away from my patients felt like eternity. At least there was an end in sight.

8-12

> Twitching thumbs. Remnants of a moment
> so golden and so pure.
> Shadows of a light so bright
> Casting away the veils of illusion.
> The shadows remain.
> The sun has set again.
> forty-one and a half years it took it to rise.
> How long before
> I see the light again?
> Twitching thumbs
> Hold my hands
> reminding me
> The sun never sets forever.

August 12, 1998

Dear Oregon Board of Medical Examiners,

This letter is to confirm that I desire and look forward to returning to my practice of medicine. My colleagues and support staff continue to share with me that my patients keep asking when I will return. I look forward to being able to let them know that I will be returning soon, and just when

Chapter 12: Diagnosis #2

that will be. With regards to my mental competence, I feel as fully competent as any practitioner could feel being out of practice for several months. I have never felt that I was not mentally competent, though I certainly agree that some of my comments to patients were inappropriate, and my charting sometimes incomplete.

As far as a treatment plan, I concur with my psychiatrist, Dr. Paltrow, and will continue to work with my therapist.

Thank you for your concerns about me, my patients, and my practice.

Sincerely,
Harriet Cohen MD

Wanting to ensure that this letter reached the hands of the Board as timely as possible, I drove downtown and hand carried it, along with the confidentiality releases, to the office of the Board. I could feel my heart beating more forcefully than usual, but my fears were partly reassured by my thumbs, which had found another great parking space just outside the building.

So this was where they made all their decisions about me. It was conservatively tidy in grays and soft greens. Nice, but not ostentatious.

I walked through the heavy door leading into the office of the Board and smiled at the clerk. "I have a letter that Ms. Wong needs to receive today. Should I just leave it with you?"

"I'll make sure she gets it," replied the clerk.

Two days later my letter was answered with the following:

August 14, 1998
DELIVERED BY FACSIMILE

Thomas McDermott
Lindsay, Hart, Neil and Weigler, LLP
1300 SW Fifth Ave., Suite 3400
Portland, OR 97201

Ghostwoman

Dear Mr. McDermott,

This morning Dr. Cohen dropped off her signed releases for records and reports from Kenneth Paltrow, MD, E. K., MD, and David Bice, Ph.D. She left before I had a chance to meet with her.

Unfortunately, a misunderstanding about the due date of Dr. Cohen's records require that I will fax the releases and subpoenas to these providers today. Hopefully, Dr. Paltrow and Dr. Bice will be able to provide their records by Monday afternoon so that the interview of Dr. Cohen on September 24th may be tentatively scheduled.

Before any interview of a licensee regarding mental health issues, the case is reviewed and discussed by members of the Investigative Committee, as well as the Board's psychiatric consultant, medical director, and assistant attorney general. Before the case on Dr. Cohen can be placed on the agenda for September 3rd meeting, her file must have records from these providers for review.

The deadline for agenda items is Tuesday, August 18th; thus, my request earlier this week for Dr. Cohen's records at least a few days prior to this date. All case files are then mailed out on Wednesday and Thursday, August 19th and 20th, to the five Board members who sit on the Investigative Committee. This fixed, two-week agenda schedule has been in place for many years at the Board, and I recognize the difficulties in compiling her file on such short notice.

My supervisor, Mitchell Herman, chief investigator, and I are eager to place Dr. Cohen's case on the agendas for both September Committee meetings. My letter to Dr. Cohen requesting a response to the allegations was hand delivered to her on May 21st. Thank you for contacting Dr. Cohen's providers about expecting subpoenas and releases. Please call if you have any questions.

    Sincerely,
    Marie Wong
    Investigator

Chapter 12: Diagnosis #2

Thomas called me as soon as he received this fax, which was not until late Friday afternoon. Why weren't we advised earlier of such a time crunch for a late September meeting? Had I just wasted the last month-and-a-half seeing a psychiatrist, taking tests and getting a report written? We had complied with their every wish and now we were being told that my hearing was likely to be postponed if they could not receive my patient records from my therapist and psychiatrist by the following Monday. This was a new request. And the confidentiality of my records was supposed to be protected by law. Such protection was part of what the Board was there to advocate for!

Frantically, I placed calls to both of my doctors, who were able to have the documents copied and in the hands of the Board by the following Tuesday morning. Again, I hand carried them.

Another request came in for a note from Dr. Bice stating my treatment plan. Again I hand carried it to the Board to make the deadline.

'Problem: Issues of sadness and unresolved grief re: life experiences.
Treatment: Regular therapy appointments with focus on resolving grief issues.'

Chapter 13
New Demands

8-17

    today... Dr. Bice-- discussion of why I keep seeing him, where the sadness comes from. He asked how things were going with Frank. Not much different, sometimes he's kind, but not affectionate. And the other day he got so angry with me for beating him home from our kayaking trip when I took a side street through the neighborhood. He was more concerned for the neighborhood than for Iyra and I to get home in time for her Hebrew lesson.
    Dr. Bice believes I intellectualize and don't allow my feelings. I say I allow. I do, just privately. Then they pass.
    But I'm not sure I know where my feelings come from.
    It looks like they come from outside of me, but

Chapter 13: New Demands

the teachers in my books say otherwise. And I do often notice a sadness that wells from within, waking up sad some days, waking up happy on other ones.

Where does the water from the well come from? Inside, outside, everything is so connected.

Discussion of patients' rights. Confidentiality issues. Dr. Bice is so protective. Says they have no right to ask for his notes. He's afraid I'll let them do what they will with me and not fight for my license or my rights. I assure him not so, I earned my degree and did nothing to violate it. I would not have been granted it if it was not important for me to have. I just don't have the energy to fight every issue.

It's odd how discussing my legal hassles never brings up an emotional response the way talking about my need for nurturing does. All Dr. Bice or Dr. Paltrow need to do is mention that subject and I explode into an unstoppable convulsion of tears.

Needing nurturing. I can barely say those words without feeling my throat close up.

I did manage to bring it up to Frank the other day. Told him how emotional it was for me to acknowledge my own nurturing needs and how good it felt when he made me lunch last Friday. Then something shifted for a while— he was so much more giving and loving, he was such a dear.

And then we go back to being who we're used to being.

The sunset is beautiful. Purple clouds edged in luminous pink.

Robin and family and Jacob were over for lunch. I made blueberry pancakes. Robin sculpted melon balls. We feasted on good food and friendship. She's so beautiful, that Robin and her family.

They all joined Jade and I at a political forum. I wanted to ask the Senator about his miserable farm-workers legislation, but he completely sidestepped the question, wanting to focus only on senior issues. The kids compelled us to leave soon after that. It's so weird how a politician I agree with on so many issues, can initiate such a thoughtless piece of legislation.

Ms. Wong returned my call at 6:30. She's just trying to make sure I get on the interview schedule for Sept. 24th. She said she'd accept my note from Dr. Bice.

I went off about my right of privacy, and she recommended I talk to my lawyer about it. I guess I am a little angry about it after all.

* * * * *

The following week I received a call from Thomas. Ms. Wong had contacted him and relayed that the Investigative Committee (I.C.) was requesting an independent evaluation by a psychiatrist of their choosing. They'd given him three names to choose from.

"WHAT??!!! But I called them before I set up my appointment with Dr. Paltrow for just this reason! They assured me that Dr. Paltrow was in good standing with the Board. Why wasn't his an independent opinion?"

Thomas shared my infuriation, but reminded me it was still in my best interest to go along with it.

I hung up, seething, and called Dr. Paltrow's office to

Chapter 13: New Demands

ask whether he had heard of any of the names I was given. I first spoke with his secretary, Jean, and she could hear the irritation in my voice, rising with intensity as I explained my situation.

Jean calmly reminded me that the connections that we make along the way can be more important than where we think we are going. Then she assured me she'd run the list by Dr. Paltrow as soon as he was done with his patient and get back to me as soon as possible.

It was not more than an hour before the phone rang. The only name that Dr. Paltrow was familiar with was Dr. Westman, and from what he knew of him, he thought he would be fine.

I wanted this over with, hung up and called Dr. Westman immediately, hoping somehow to meet the almost impossible deadline I thought I had on the 24th. Early that afternoon Dr. Westman returned my call.

His voice was deep and pleasant, and he was quite respectful as I shared the nature of the evaluation I needed. I told him very briefly about my spiritual experience and asked if he thought such an experience was necessarily pathological. He did not, so I scheduled the soonest appointment with him, September 8th, and tried to relax into a soft belly breath as I hung up the phone.

Two days later Thomas left me another voice mail. Ms. Wong had called him to let us know that the I.C. had changed their mind. Only one of the physicians, Dr. Thompson, would suffice.

I stormed back and forth through the small kitchen, scowling at the cabinets, then quickly dialed Thomas back, as it was late on a Friday afternoon and I didn't know how long he would be in his office. "I'm glad you're still in. I just got your message, and what they want is totally unacceptable! How can they limit me to *one* psychiatrist in all of Portland and call that an independent evaluation?"

I could hear his own anger. "I completely agree with you. And I have no idea why they're being so unreasonable. I've worked with them on a number of cases, and I've never had them do this before."

"I already made an appointment this morning with Dr. Westman for the 8th." I paused a moment to collect my thoughts. "What I'd like you to do is to contact the investigative committee and let them know this. Then can you see if they'll accept it?"

"I'll do what I can."

"They can't force me to see one specific person, can they?"

"Probably not. But like I've said, they can drag this whole process out for months. I've seen them do that. The more we cooperate with them, the faster we can get you back to work."

"I'd like that. But you know what else I want? I want you to write them a letter laying out the way they've been stringing me along. If they wanted me to see someone in particular they had no business waiting a month after they received Dr. Paltrow's report to let me know this. I don't know what I'll do with it, but I'd like the documentation."

"I'll be more than happy to write that letter!"

Thomas' sympathetic ear diffused my rage. By the time I hung up, it had dwindled to a simmer.

Nothing more that I can do about it now, I thought, and headed upstairs for a short meditation before fixing dinner.

Sitting on my pillows, I put my attention, one by one, on all the parts of my body, consciously trying to relax my muscles. Then I began my focused breathing, beginning in my belly. It was hard to keep my thoughts and my anger at the Board from resurfacing, so I put my attention on that for a while, and observed how it felt: the tension in my neck and my face, the belly that couldn't seem to remember to stay soft, the headache from the tension in my scalp. I reminded myself things were still in God's

Chapter 13: New Demands

hands. Thumb twitched "yes" without my even asking. And I began to appreciate the experience as an opportunity for self-growth, for learning to speak up for myself, finding the joy, the dance in jumping through all the hoops and trying to connect with the hoop holders in a gracious way.

In the middle of dinner preparations the phone rang.

"Harriet?" It was Theresa, my clinic manager. "I'm just getting to my mail and there's a letter for you marked 'Confidential, URGENT, Open Immediately'. It's from the Board."

Why would the Board send important papers to my work where I am not allowed to be?

I asked Theresa to open it and read it to me. The papers were notification of the process, and an application for having my license reinstated. It would take a minimum of three to four weeks *after* my interview with the investigative committee before I could return to work.

"Looks like it'll be longer than I thought before I can come back. I'm really sorry. I know it's a problem for the clinic to be covering my schedule with on-call physicians."

"Don't worry about the clinic, we'll make do. Greg is doing fine with your patients. I'm just sorry you're having to go through such a mess. "

In my yoga class, I watched my progress change after each surprise that the Board threw to me. My one-legged postures that had been balanced, suddenly toppled in seconds. Even my strength seemed to be affected and I'd have to pull out of postures earlier than usual, heart beating and sweat pouring after very little time. Still, yoga was one of the stabilizing beacons in my life, as were my friends, old and new.

I met Laurie one night at a different synagogue that had more of a mystical focus, where I'd gone looking for some spiritual camaraderie. The Rabbi was talking about

Ghostwoman

loving thy neighbor as thyself. I piped in about the importance of "self" in that equation only to discover, that was the focus of the discussion before my late arrival. Laurie made similar comments during the discussion and we exchanged phone numbers after the service.

I stumbled across her number months later and we finally got together over a cup of tea. Having connected over each other's comments, it was not too surprising to discover that, like me, she'd had an experience of unitive consciousness and longed for the opportunity to talk about her experience with someone who could somewhat understand it.

She was intelligent, compassionate, and spontaneous.

"I knew we had something very deep, in common," she said, after we'd shared our stories. Then she leaned a bit closer. "But in addition to my unitive experience, I've also been treated for bipolar disease, and there's quite a difference! With one is the feeling of wholeness, healing and functioning totally in sync with yourself and with others. The disease is nothing like that at all. And I know what you mean about losing your credibility. Sometimes it still frightens me to tell people about my illness."

Laurie's mystical experience was similar in many ways to my own. The Oneness with All sounded the same, the feeling of profound love for all was the same, and a major disruption in one's life beforehand was also a familiar theme. In Laurie's case it was the diagnosis of a very malignant form of cancer that I'd been taught was almost universally fatal that was part of the trigger for her experience. But here she was, years later, with the cancer nowhere to be found.

Sept. 14, 1998
Personal and Confidential
Harriet Cohen, MD

Chapter 13: New Demands

Dear Dr. Cohen,

This letter memorializes messages I left for you and your attorney, Thomas McDermott, on September 4, 1998, regarding your return to practice.

Members of the Investigative Committee discussed your case at its monthly meeting on Sept. 3, 1998, and the matter remains open. The Committee requests that you seek a psychiatric evaluation by L. Thompson, MD.
Only Dr. Thompson will suffice, and I apologize for any inconvenience that this request has caused. The Committee plans to interview you, but only after Dr. Thompson's assessment is completed and her report furnished to Board members for review. Unfortunately, an interview with the committee on September 24th is not feasible. One will be arranged after Dr. Thompson's report is received. The Committee meets once a month, and the next meetings are scheduled for November 5 and December 3.

To arrange an appointment, Dr Thompson can be reached at _____ and her office is located at _____. It is essential that you notify me of the time and date of the evaluation so that pertinent information can be provided to Dr. Thompson. She will need to furnish the Board with a copy of your evaluation and diagnostic conclusions, so you must sign a release allowing her to send her report to the Board. Any cost incurred regarding the assessment and evaluation is the responsibility of you, the licensee under investigation.

You or Mr. McDermott may call me if you have any questions. Again, thank you for your cooperation and time. I recognize that such delays can be frustrating.

Sincerely,
Marie Wong
Investigator

cc: Thomas McDermott, attorney
      Mitchell Herman, chief investigator

    The postponement of my interview felt like an eternity. I read the letter with a great heaviness, then became infuriated over the need the Board had to somehow alert Dr. Thompson about me before my appointment. What kind of "pertinent information" were they talking about?

I remembered a study I'd read about in Dr. Kaplan's book that illustrated the effect of suggestion on a clinician's opinion of whether they are looking at psychopathology.

In this study, psychologists wrote a script of a diagnostic interview of a functional, expressive, "normal" man. They had a professional actor play the part of this interviewee in a way that was intended to demonstrate a lack of psychological problems, but rather an intellectual curiosity about therapy.

They taped this interview, then showed the tape to the undergraduates and psychology students, casually remarking that the person on the tape "looked neurotic, but was actually psychotic." A group of psychiatrists were told that two psychiatry Board members had agreed that the man looked neurotic, but was actually psychotic. All viewers were asked how the interviewee should be classified, choosing from a list that included a variety of mental disorders, personality types, and the classification of normal, or healthy personality.

Significant numbers of evaluators diagnosed the man as psychotic, and most of those who did not said he was neurotic. Only a tiny percentage of evaluators classified the man as healthy, normal, or even having a "mild adjustment disorder," and none of these evaluators were the psychiatrists.

As a control group, the experiment was repeated three times. In the first group the prestigious person showing the film said that the patient "looked like a normal healthy man." In the second group, no prior suggestion at all was made. And in the third group, the patient was taken out of the clinical setting and the same interview was done as a personnel interview for

Chapter 13: New Demands

employment, to select engineers and scientists for a research corporation. The tape was modified minimally for this last group.

Not a single member of any of these last three groups considered the man to be psychotic. Most classified him either as normal, or as having "mild adjustment problems."

Mon. Sept. 14

I did the three-Rune reading this morning.
Where I am now— Opening.
The problem I need to overcome— Possessions.
The goal— Wholeness.

What sort of possessions do I need to let go of? Is it possessions in general? Or is it my license to practice medicine? Or is it simply the characteristic of possessiveness, needing to work on non-attachment and letting go? I ask my thumbs and they are clear that I'm not to let go of my license. That's not surprising, I received too much cosmic assistance getting through medical school for it to have been unnecessary.

Thank you.

Sept. 15

Robert Gray Middle School picnic behind me, Reike Elementary school picnic tonight, the *Bhagavad-Gita* before me. Dr. Bice recommended that I check it out at my last visit when I shared my confusion about how to deal with the issues my life has laid out before me.

When do we fight? When do we not let go?
The library didn't have either of the versions

Ghostwoman

that Dr. Bice had recommended, but the one they had looks interesting. *The Bhagavad-Gita As It Is*. It has the Sanskrit letters, followed by the transliteration with English equivalents, the translation, followed by a lengthy commentary. It reminds me of the way the Torah is dissected. I believe these two sacred texts were both written/passed down about the same time. Another interesting feature they share is in the Preface of this version of the *Gita*. The Swami writing the commentary describes the *Gita* using the same metaphor as the Torah: an upside down tree of life, the branches extending into the earth, and the roots extending into heaven.

I've read that even the languages were created similarly— monosyllable root words modified by prefixes and suffixes.

I've been taken off the September 24th schedule. The Board didn't think that I could be seen and have a report ready by then. They should know. They limited me to one psychiatrist in all of Portland and may as well have a handle on her schedule.

I consult my Runes again. Upside down Possessions.

Out of all the 25 possibilities, Possessions comes up again. The upside down meaning:

"There may be considerable frustration in your life if you draw *Fehu* reversed, a wide variety of dispossessions ranging from trivial to severe. You fall short in your efforts; you reach out and miss; you are compelled to

Chapter 13: New Demands

stand by and watch helplessly while what you've gained dwindles away. Observe what is happening. Examine these events from an open perspective and ask, "What do I need to learn from this in my life?"

Even if there is occasion for joy, do not let yourself be seduced into mindless joyousness. Reversed, this Rune indicates that doubtful situations are abundant and come in many forms and guises. Here you are being put in touch with the shadow side of possessions. Yet, all this is part of coming-to-be and passing-away, and not that which abides. In dealing with the shadow side of *Fehu*, you have an opportunity to recognize where your true nourishment lies."

(from *The Book of Runes*, by Ralph H. Blum)

Frank was in the garden spreading bark dust. He'd already done all the weeding and planting and setting up a drip sprinkler system. My leg was better, but it wasn't up to the rigors of pushing on a shovel. And my right knee still couldn't bend well enough to make squatting in the garden any fun.

"Hi," I smiled and gave him a kiss. "You're too sweaty for a hug."

He smiled broadly and there was an excitement in his eyes. "Come around back and tell me what you think of the rope ladder."

A few days before, Frank had come home with a massive spool of inch and a half thick rope. He'd been experimenting with tying it in different ways to make a rope ladder for our tree house, a platform about one-and-a-half stories up in our walnut tree. It was otherwise only reachable by climbing through the branches of the laurel trees that grew beneath it.

Using the leftover redwood from building our deck at the other house, Frank had completely rebuilt the rotting structure that came with the house. He climbed through the laurel branches carrying his tools and the

Ghostwoman

wood, and somehow propped up himself and the wood by using the original tree house platform. The kids said that the new structure was beautiful, but I was still very anxious about Jade's friends climbing up the dangerous ascent that was required to reach it, not to mention the potential for easily falling from a platform so high in the tree. I'd already had to rescue one stranded child with the extension ladder. That was when Frank set to the task of creating a climbing structure out of thick rigging rope, with some ropes around the periphery of the platform to make it safer.

"Wow!" Stable rigging was tied through the laurel trees from the ground on up to the tree house in huge evenly-spaced knots. It was a giant macramé, all one piece of rope and all connected with living branches.

"Go ahead, give it a try!" he said.

Hand by hand, left leg always leading right, I climbed the rope creation that was ever so much easier than a ladder. "It's wonderful!" Up I climbed until my head could peer over the top of the platform for the first time. Glowing redwood boards of varying widths created a brilliant floor in the canopy of the walnut tree. I was the eyes of the tree, and out beyond was a wonderful sweeping view of the valley below.

My fear of heights wouldn't allow me to make the last ascent over the top of the rope and onto the platform, just yet. I enjoyed the view from my more stable position. Enjoyed, too, the good feelings between Frank and me that moment, as things between us had continued to be difficult, making moments of connection particularly precious.

Frank surrounds himself with tangible things. He builds and creates things that we can enjoy for years. I, however, am wanting only to surround myself with books. It is like I'm in school again, reading

Chapter 13: New Demands

so many different books at once. Only this time, I've chosen them all. The *Bhagavad-Gita* is a little chewy and is taking awhile. *Mutant Message Down Under*, on the other hand, was downed in a few days. Even Frank liked that one; it's the first book we've shared in years.

Sept. 26.

"Born to be Wiiiild!..... Like a true nature's child..." I rock out to the radio while baking four loaves of zucchini bread from the zucchini we have grown in the garden.

"So I want to be a paper back writer.!..."

The piles in my office multiplied over the weekend. Cleaning off my desk, I turned three piles into five large ones... and I want to read to Jade up in the tree house, having conquered the last step of actually climbing off that wonderfully secure ladder.... The day is warm and sunny. But the laundry pile is mountainous.

I hear, and read, and believe that art, using the right side of the brain, nurtures intuition. My goal— to draw or paint twice a week. It has been two weeks since I have found the time to touch anything.

The radio sang on... "Yes it's the same kind of story that seems to come from a long time ago... There's no explaining the imagination....."

"Come along if you can to the magic side of your mind....."

Chapter 14
Four More Opinions

By the middle of the month, my lawyers' bills were over $700, and it was clear that I was nowhere near finished with this mess. The unpaid psychiatric bills were close to a thousand, and my insurance had reached its limit. Before the accident I had never had a lawyer. Now I had two: one to deal with the accident (which was in a waiting phase and required little energy or investment of either time or emotion), and one to deal with the Board.

At the end of the month my disability insurance carrier added its own conclusion to my situation. They had reviewed all the documents and were pleased to inform me that my request for disability benefits had been approved. I was to be paid sixty percent of my basic monthly earnings, for the period of time up until August fifth, the date that Dr. Paltrow completed his report and sent it in to the Board, advising that I was competent to return to work. It was their feeling that I had been misdiagnosed, and since their coverage was only for medical disability, not bureaucratic or political ones, there would be no compensation beyond that date.

Chapter 14: Four Moe Opinions

Thomas spoke with me over the phone about the letter. "I think we can argue the case with the disability insurance. You're still unable to work because of the diagnosis."

"Thomas, if we argue for me to get further disability payments, we're arguing that I'm disabled. No. I want to let it go. I agree with them."

_____**Oregon** Board of Medical Examiners
620 Crown Plaza
1500 SW First Avenue
Portland, Or 97201-5826
September 28, 1998

Mr. Thomas E. McDermott
Lindsay Hart Neil & Weigler, LLP

Re: Harriet Cohen, MD

Dear Mr. McDermott:

Your letter to Dr. Heusch dated September 24, 1998 was referred to me since it relates to a matter currently under investigation. I reviewed the implications and allegations contained in your letter against the case record. We could clearly get into a lengthy discussion about demands versus the orderly gathering of information sufficient for the Board of Medical Examiners to reach a proper decision, as well as communication.

However, at this point I do not think that meets the best interest of the Board or your client. I will place your concerns, as well as your request, for the Board to accept an evaluation from Dr. Westman on the agenda for the November 5, 1998 Investigative Committee. If you have additional information you wish the IC to consider, communicate it to Ms. Wong and we will bring it to the attention of the IC as well. The IC will decide how it wants to proceed with the case.

Ghostwoman

If you have any questions or wish to discuss the matter further, feel free to call me at 503/229-5770.

Sincerely,
Mitchell Herman
Chief Investigator

By the time I had received this information, I already had my appointment with Dr. Westman. He had a small office without a receptionist. A sign instructed me to have a seat.

I breathed consciously while nervously waiting. Soft belly. Trust the process. The door to the waiting room opened and a large, clean shaven man with a jolly, round face came out and greeted me. Following him into a small office, I sat in a comfortable chair facing him and began to relay my story. Having recently read Dr. Cheek's book on hypnotherapy, I felt a little more comfortable describing my thumb phenomena in clinical terms, which sounded less delusional even to me.

Dr. Westman listened quietly, interjecting questions as needed, to do the evaluation. He did not say anything that made me think that he believed that my experience was pathological. "You speak very clearly," was the only specific comment that I can remember.

"Only sometimes," I'd answered. "I am just as often at a loss for words, unable to think of the right thing to say until at least thirty minutes or so later."

The interview took little more than an hour. We shook hands and I left.

A big waste of time, I thought to myself after receiving the response of Mr. Herman. I'd have to wait at least another month just to get them to discuss accepting Dr. Westman's report! I felt defeated and asked my thumbs if it was in our best interest to schedule an appointment with Dr. Linda Thompson.

She returned my call the same day and was very kind over the phone. She found an appointment time for me as quickly as possible so that I could have the report in time for the November IC meeting.

Yom Kippur, the holiest day of the Jewish Year, began at sundown the following day. As I worked in the kitchen on the holiday feast that would prepare us for our twenty-four hour fast, Iyra came into the room. "Mom, the basement is full of water," she said.

"What do you mean the basement is full of water?" I followed her down the stairs and though not exactly flooded, there was a slow but steady stream of water coming in from the far wall. It cascaded across the cement floor, then funneled down the drain in the middle of the room.

Frank came home from work about then and looked at the little creek that was running through the house. He quickly figured out that we had a broken water main and turned off all the water. This would be a challenge for the dozen guests I'd invited the following afternoon, who were joining us for a potluck to break our day of prayer and fasting.

I came home early from services the next day so that I could put together an apple crisp from our abundant apple tree crop. As soon as I placed the crisp in the oven, the oven stopped working.

Happy New Year!

October 1

The futility of life... raising children, loving children, teaching children, and being there, while the world suffers in hate and intolerance.

While I, wanting to learn, wanting to help, am shackled by my slowness and a memory that refuses to believe that it exists. So many books, so little time... dreams... how to live with a heart, through heart. A heart dissected by conflict with authority, broken pipes, broken oven, and picking up after kids and being ears that listen to them all— all the time. So it sometimes seems.

A morning of internal torment takes its yoga class and opens its shoulders for the first time!

Arching backwards, my hands meet heels after months of flapping in the breeze and grasping at the air,

Find their mark!
Heels, so close and so hard to reach
until five months later
connection is made.
When we keep trying and
keep believing in ourselves,
and have patience,
Connection happens.

October 6th I had my appointment with Dr. Thompson. She sent me a card beforehand with the appointment time and directions. Her thoughtfulness helped me get over the resentment I had about being there at all. She was a nice-looking woman with gray hair and a loose-fitting, conservative dress. She looked to be in her fifties, and her manner was professional and aloof, yet kind. I asked her about her personal views on spirituality. She shared that part of her education occurred in a Catholic teaching institution, but that was all.

After almost an hour-and-a-half, we hadn't finished the interview, so we scheduled a follow-up visit. I brought up the time constraint, as I understood it from Ms. Wong's letter to me— that the Board needed to have the report in their hands two weeks before the interview date, at the very latest. Dr. Thompson was grateful for this information, as she had not been made aware of any time

Chapter 14: Four Moe Opinions

issues. She made a place for me two days later at 6:10 pm, after she had finished with her day's already full schedule. I was most grateful to her for making this accommodation on my behalf, and I left her with a copy of my personal response to Dr. Eugene's report. I figured the Board had sent her his evaluation, and I wanted to balance it with my own version of that interview and my experience. We shook hands and I left.

At my second visit, Dr. Thompson concurred with the opinions of Dr. Paltrow and Mr. McDermott regarding my written response. "I wouldn't recommend giving this to the Board either. They wouldn't understand it," she said. Then we focused on the remaining questions she needed me to answer.

At the end of my visit I brought out Dr. Gersten's book, *Are You Getting Enlightened or Losing Your Mind?* "It's written by a psychiatrist who's very familiar with spiritual experiences and successfully integrates spiritual counseling into his practice. I don't know whether you're interested or not, but you're welcome to borrow it if you'd like."

She politely turned down the opportunity. Then, since time was so tight, she agreed to send her report to me at the same time she would send it to the Board. If I had disagreement with anything in the report, I could schedule an appointment with her to discuss it, but the original version would be in the hands of the Board in time for me to get on the November schedule, and it had been her experience that they would accept a clarification that came shortly thereafter.

The leaves turned brilliant colors as I waited for a hearing with the Board. Time puttered along with swim meets and Hebrew lessons for Iyra, after-school art classes and Shabbat School for Jade, music lessons for both, community meetings, and the plumbing job from hell that lasted almost the entire month. The plumber had gone

Ghostwoman

through more than I had since I'd last seen him. He looked like he was in congestive heart failure. I couldn't fire him, though, he needed the job too badly.

"Have you seen a doctor lately?"

"No... I'm fine," he said, catching his breath at the top of the stairs, his face all ashen and drawn.

"Looks like you might have some heart trouble."

"No, I don't have time to see a doctor. I've got two granddaughters to take care of. Besides, I don't trust doctors."

"I can understand. I'm a doctor."

He smiled slightly, in appreciation of my attempt to empathize. "My daughter had cancer. They said she'd have a good chance if she took chemo. But they gave her too much and she was dead in two days. That's why I'm raising her kids."

Some days, the plumber and I would just sit outside on the deck and talk while we waited for his less-than-reliable assistant to show up. He was always so apologetic about how long it was taking to get the job done.

"As long as you've got us hooked up to water, we're fine. I'm just sorry it's turned into such a miserable job for you," I said.

He wondered what kind of a doctor I was, and where I worked, so I told him why I wasn't working.

"I used to be a spiritual man myself. Then one thing after another happened. Lost my daughter, lost another son, then Bill got in that terrible accident. It's hard to keep your faith."

Occasionally I'd make it over to the old Wholeness Center on Wednesday nights, where a wonderful group of people would congregate over a vegetarian dinner in my old kitchen, discussing all sorts of alternative healing modalities.

It was a well-read group of creative folks, and it was here that I was given the name of Stanislav Grof, a pioneer

Chapter 14: Four Moe Opinions

psychiatrist in the field of transpersonal consciousness. He'd been exploring the therapeutic value of non-ordinary states of consciousness for over three decades, and clarified how spiritual experiences differed from mental illness.

Spiritual Emergency: When Personal Transformation Becomes a Crisis. In this book, a series of essays by psychiatrists in the field of transpersonal experiences, a recurring theme was that spiritual, and/or mystical experiences differed significantly from mental illness.

Spiritual emergence was characterized by: 1) most often a sincere involvement in meditation, and/or other forms of spiritual practice; 2) emergence from these unusual states of mind into a sense of greater well-being, *higher functioning in daily life*, stability, and in many cases, healing of long-standing emotional, spiritual or physical problems; and 3) therapeutic need for support and understanding of the spiritual emergence process.

In contrast, mental illness is characterized by: 1) somewhat predictable patterns of illness development within age ranges and genetic families (though recent literature suggests this is controversial); 2) persistence of an unstable mind and personality which greatly limits the functioning in daily life; and 3) requirement of suppressive therapy to help enable the individual to function toward his/ her desired potential.

Spiritual Emergency, by Stanislav and Christina Grof. And where did I think I would put it? The books in the office are two deep, where there's room. Magazines are stashed on the tops of the books. I've moved a few armloads of things I won't need down to the basement shelves. I hate to do that. The wood on the back is cracked and warped like it gets damp down there.

Ghostwoman

My kitchen desk now has a whole row of my ongoing readers lined up. I'm a third of the way through the hypnosis text, then there's Carl Jung's book, *The Archetypes of the Collective Unconscious*, waiting for me, the large text, *Zen and the Brain*, which arrived last week and I haven't even opened yet. And the bookstore caught me again. What do they put in the air that makes me always walk out with something? *Stumbling Toward Enlightenment*, by Larkin, *When Things Fall Apart*, by Pema Chodron. My yoga magazine rolls in monthly before I've finished the last one. And the Institute of Noetic Sciences magazine that I just began to get is wonderful— Scientists studying consciousness!

Then there's *Alternative Therapies* with an article by Dr. Dossey that I always look forward to. I wonder what the Board would think of my choice in journals these days? Yes, your honor, I keep up with my journal reading....

By October 17th, I received Dr. Thompson's report. It is interesting to me that now, over two years later, I can read it and feel the compassion and work that went into writing the seven-and-a-half page, single-spaced report. At the time I received it, however, I remember feeling happy only because it was done, which meant that I would be on the schedule for an interview with the IC on the 5th of November. Otherwise, it irritated me. I focused on the numerous minor errors in the narrative of the sequence of events of my life, and also had issues with Dr. Thompson's assessment and plan. It was better than Eugene's, whose prognosis requiring lithium had already been disproved over time, but it was not what I had hoped for.

Chapter 14: Four Moe Opinions

It included my history leading up to the mystical experience, the experience, and the immediate events that followed including the evaluations with Drs. Eugene and Paltrow. Dr. Thompson also summarized all the documents: the memo from Dr. Charleston, the letter from Dr. Eugene to Dr. Charleston, records from Dr. Bice, and Dr. Paltrow. Her assessments were as follows:

MENTAL STATUS EXAMINATION

On both occasions Dr. Cohen was seen, she presented as a slender, athletic appearing, dark-haired woman who was casually attired and had given good attention to hygiene, modesty, and details of grooming. Her manner was socially appropriate, direct, and open, if somewhat cautious initially. She made good eye contact. Mood was neither depressed nor euphoric and included anger/frustration at her licensing difficulties and at what she sees as Dr, Eugene's misdiagnosis. Affect was appropriate to mood and thought content. Speech and motor activity were normal. There was no disorder of thought form. Thought content included non-delusional interest in spirituality and healing. Dr. Cohen was also invested in interpreting her April 1998 experience as spiritual RATHER THAN manic. Judgment and insight were good. Dr. Cohen related to the possibility of discussing her April experience with a BMA committee, expressed a strong commitment to personal integrity, especially regarding her intention of voicing her truth regarding her spiritual experience. There was no evidence of risk of harm or of psychiatric impairment of medical judgment.

ASSESSMENT

Dr. Cohen has experienced catastrophic levels of stress in the past year, however we psychiatrically label her prolonged tearfulness in 1997 and her spiritual experience in 1998. Beyond noting this overriding contextual observation, I will list below what I see as important elements in Dr. Cohen's history and then will discuss diagnostic possibilities and suggestions.
1. Dr. Cohen agrees that her behavior was euphoric and unusual for her in April 1998 when her supervisor received complaints about her. She readily describes her 1997

Ghostwoman

emotional and physical traumas and her two months of related sadness.

2. Dr. Cohen's supervisor has documented that Dr. Cohen's interpersonal judgment was impaired with patients and that her clinical documentation was inadequate in April 1998. No medical harm was done by Dr. Cohen.
3. Dr. Cohen has throughout viewed her April 1998 experience as spiritual, valuable, and life-enhancing. She has consistent language for discussing this experience. There is a religious and medical subculture from which this language derives.
4. Dr. Charleston saw Dr. Cohen during the April experience and considered the possibility of psychiatric disorder as an explanation. She was acting as Dr. Cohen's clinical supervisor, not her physician.
5. Dr. Bice saw Dr. Cohen five days before the April experience and about a week after it ended. He interpreted Dr. Cohen's experience as dissociative in nature.
6. Dr. Eugene first met Dr. Cohen about two weeks after the April experience ended. He interpreted her efforts to educate him about spirituality as residuals of a manic episode, though he documented that she was neither depressed nor euphoric then. He recommended mood-stabilizing medical treatment and cautioned against psychotherapy. Prognosticly, he saw Dr. Cohen as likely to recover fully and return to practice.
7. Dr. Paltrow first met Dr. Cohen about six weeks after the April experience ended. Screening psychological testing then showed no major pathology. Dr Paltrow and Dr. Cohen agreed on a bereavement interpretation of her 1997 sadness. Dr Cohen experienced benefit from her work with Dr. Paltrow and has voluntarily returned to treatment with him.
8. I first met Dr. Cohen about six months after the April experience ended. Her mental status then was remarkable only for anger and frustration at interpretations of her and at her licensing difficulties. She also saw the issues related to her April experience in a dichotomized manner... as though spiritual and psychiatric labels were mutually exclusive.
9. Dr. Cohen has no history of diagnosed psychiatric disorder or psychiatric treatment prior to late 1997. She had some euphoric behavior on high doses of steroids several years ago (treatment for a serious platelet disorder). She

Chapter 14: Four Moe Opinions

had no postpartum depression with her first two pregnancies. She has no family history of mood disorder or psychotic disorder. She had no previous professional difficulties.

Before I discuss possible psychiatric formulations for Dr. Cohen's experiences, I want to make a comment about Dr. Cohen's spiritual interpretation of her April experience. I think her current interpretation is logically consistent and meaningful to her. I accept that she had a spiritual experience.

There seems to be some dispute among evaluators about whether or how Dr. Cohen's spiritual experience might ALSO be labeled psychiatrically, and Dr. Cohen has objected to psychiatric labeling of the experience. All evaluators have proposed reasonable possible diagnostic considerations. None of the evaluators' arguments appears to me conclusive.

It is clear that Dr. Cohen was low in mood in late 1997, but several of her physical symptoms suggestive of depression were also attributable to her physical condition. The DSM-IV label for low mood in the context of physical illness which might mimic some symptoms is "depression not otherwise specified." Although I would agree that Dr. Cohen was bereaved as well when she was crying for those eight weeks, I would not see her 1997 sadness as <u>uncomplicated</u> bereavement.

It is clear that Dr. Cohen was euphoric and altered in her medical judgment for at least 10-14 days in April 1998. Dr. Paltrow's arguments against the period's meeting full criteria for a manic episode are consistent with the history Dr. Cohen gave me. Without a full manic or mixed episode, a Bipolar I Disorder diagnosis cannot be made. "Mood disorder not otherwise specified" might appropriately label our uncertainty regarding the prognostic significance of the euphoric experience. I would not argue with Dr Bice's interpretation of Dr Cohen's experience as dissociative... but I think the only DSM-IV label applicable would be "dissociative disorder not otherwise specified."

Although none of these "not otherwise specified" diagnosis

Ghostwoman

provided prognostic assistance for Dr. Cohen, we do have substantial information related to her prognosis. Dr. Cohen is currently without psychiatric disorder, despite her lack of the medication that Dr. Eugene recommended. She had a good premorbid psychiatric history. She has good social support. She has no family history of a mood disorder. IF she has some susceptibility to mood disturbance, it has only been uncovered by severe stress.

Even without a specific psychiatric label for Dr. Cohen's April 1998 experience, and even in the face of good psychiatric prognosis overall, we should bear in mind that Dr. Cohen's interpersonal judgment was impaired in April. If Dr. Cohen were to have a similar experience in the future, she should not attempt to practice medicine during that time. I agree with Dr. Cohen's supervisor's April 1998 decision to put Dr. Cohen on administrative leave, and I agree with the guidelines for practice outlined in the supervisor's April memo.

My attempt at a DSM-IV label for Dr. Cohen's recent experiences would be:
    Axis I. Mood disorder not otherwise specified.
    Axis II. No diagnosis.
    Axis III. Distal tibia/fibula fracture with surgical repair 10/97.
    Axis IV. Death of friend, therapeutic abortion, change of residence, administrative leave from job, suspension of medical license, resolved marital difficulties.
    Axis V. GAF 75/75

SUGGESTIONS

Dr. Cohen appears to me now psychiatrically able to practice medicine and to do so within the limits described in her supervisor's April memo to her.

Because of the uncertainty, psychiatrically, of the prognostic significance of her April euphoric experience, I think Dr. Cohen should be followed with at least monthly office visits by a psychiatrist for the next year, for periodic monitoring of her mood and for rapid access to treatment, if necessary.

Chapter 14: Four Moe Opinions

I disagree with Eugene's recommendation for medication and against psychotherapy. I do not see anti-manic medication as indicated. I do think Dr. Cohen's 1997-98 experience could be appropriately processed in psychotherapy, either with the monitoring psychiatrist or with another clinician. I would be cautious about therapy including "hypnotic regression."

This concludes the report of my evaluation and recommendations for Dr. Cohen. Please let me know if additional information is needed from me.

Sincerely,
Linda Thompson, MD

"...If she has some susceptibility to mood disturbance, it has only been uncovered by severe stress..." I lingered over this passage, thinking of my current situation with the Board and my license, not having worked for so many months, the tension in my marriage, the house with all its broken this and thats, and the lawsuit that lingered in the shadows. As if I wasn't STILL under significant stress! Then I worked through the report and corrected the historical, and other objective inaccuracies, wrote down my disagreements with Dr. Thompson's assessment, and scheduled an appointment with her to discuss the issues I had with her report.

A day later I received my formal invitation for an interview with the Investigative Committee of the Board.

October 16, 1998

PERSONAL AND CONFIDENTIAL
SENT BY CERTIFIED MAIL
ARTICLE NO. Z 594 244 813

Harriet Cohen, MD
Dear Dr. Cohen:

Ghostwoman

The Board of Medical Examiners respectfully requests your presence for an interview by a subcommittee of the Investigative Committee of the Board, pursuant to the authority outlined in ORS 677.415(1) & (4). The interview will be held at the Board's office, Suite 620 of the Crown Plaza Building, 1500 SW First Avenue, Portland, at 10:15 a.m. on Thursday, November 5, 1998.

Pursuant to 677.320(5), the current investigative summary is:

Concerns have been raised regarding your fitness to safely and competently practice medicine. The Multnomah County Department of Health placed you on administrative leave in 1998 alleging that you suffer from depression and a bipolar disorder and that you require psychiatric care and treatment.
Please come to the interview prepared to discuss the above concerns and any subsequent evaluations or treatment you may have undergone which reflect on your fitness to practice medicine.

Legally you are advised that under the provisions of ORS 677.190(23), the Board has the authority to discipline a licensee for refusing an invitation for an interview before the Investigative Committee. The Committee may ask you questions and make comments during your appearance. Please also be prepared to answer questions regarding your current workload and your continuing medical education over the last three years.

You should plan on your appearance before the committee lasting approximately 45 minutes. You have the right to be accompanied by an attorney if you so desire. Please make any request to the committee at least one week prior to the meeting for special accommodations needed for a disability or for the services of a translator due to a potential language barrier. If there is any change in the interview time and/or date, we will notify you at the earliest possible opportunity.

Please note that any supporting materials/documents that you wish to be considered by members of the investigative Committee as part of this review process must be received

Chapter 14: Four Moe Opinions

in this office no less than ten days prior to your appearance. If you have any questions concerning this matter, please feel free to contact this office.

Very truly yours,
Mitchell Herman
Chief Investigator

cc: Loren Hande, Board Counsel
Tom McDermott

Accompanying this letter to me was a standard form that gave further details regarding what I should expect at my interview.

I sat on the sofa at the end of Dr. Thompson's room for this last appointment. She sat in her chair facing me, with her desk behind her. It was a fairly large room, allowing plenty of space between us.

"I don't understand why you presume that I shouldn't practice medicine during any future experiences similar to my April experience. I fully agreed with my initial errors in my counseling and further agreed to chart in a more conventional manner. While in my altered state, I learned that I needed to be more subtle in my approach to these matters and to always come from the perspective of the patients' beliefs. No further incidents occurred during the next three days that I practiced. On the contrary, I felt like I had some breakthroughs with patients with whom I'd been getting nowhere for years. There were no bad outcomes. The only disagreement with my medical treatment recommendation was minor and controversial and I have journal articles to back me up. I was the one able to talk a patient who was having a myocardial infarction into going to the hospital, not my colleague who was seeing the patient that day.

"Perhaps instead, if I ever attain such an altered state of consciousness again, rather than prohibiting me from practice, I should be required to alert my supervisor so

Ghostwoman

that she could establish whether my practice was suffering at all, or whether, in fact, it might in some way be improved."

Dr. Thompson would not budge from her position. "The Board would never buy that," she said.

I took a breath and paused. "Dr. Thompson, are you familiar with Carl Jung's theory of the collective unconsciousness?"

She looked back at me with equal earnestness. "I've read some of Jung's work. Are you aware that many of Jung's contemporaries thought that he was schizophrenic in his later years?"

Dr. Thompson did spend some time talking about how this whole process was hurtful to me, and how the system needed to change to avoid such unnecessary harm to its physicians. She was aware of the different processes in other states that would never have allowed a situation like mine to have developed. She quickly typed up the corrections to her initial report, and had it ready for me to hand carry to the Oregon Board of Medical Examiners office the following day.

Linda M. Thompson, M.D.
Physician, Psychiatry
October 20, 1998

Edmond Deutsch, MD Chair
Oregon Board of Medical Examiners
620 Crown Plaza
1500 SW First Avenue
Portland, OR 97201

Re: Harriet Cohen, MD
Dear Dr. Heusch:

This letter is being given to Harriet Cohen, MD, to hand carry to you to be included with my October 14, 1998, psychiatric evaluation at the next Investigative Committee meeting. Dr. Cohen met with me today, at her request, to correct several errors of fact contained in my earlier report and to discuss

Chapter 14: Four Moe Opinions

her concerns regarding my recommendations.

Dr. Cohen had areas of disagreement with my recommendations for her. This letter contains corrections of my factual errors but does not alter my assessment or recommendations. Dr. Cohen has pointed out some potential for misunderstanding of my recommendations, so I will help clarify them. I will also add a final thought.

CORRECTIONS OF HISTORY
—Dr. Cohen's actual date of administrative leave was April 17, 1998
—It was Dr. Cohen's grandfather-in-law who died September 29, 1997, not her friend. Her friend was terminally ill then, and died of breast cancer in December 1997. Dr. Cohen's positive pregnancy test was about two days before the grandfather-in-law's death.
—Dr. Cohen's feelings of worthlessness in late 1997 were related to "not knowing myself" around several recent issues, not just to feelings about her gynecologic decision.
—Dr. Cohen had not yet read of "Samadhi" experiences at the time of her April change in behavior. She read of such experiences after her own experience. Herbert Benson's books are actually about relaxation through meditation.
—Dr. Cohen's medical charting during her April experience was not ONLY "for fun." She reports including pertinent clinical information but in a more relaxed way than she had done previously. She disagrees that her medical judgment was impaired.
—Dr. Cohen was not euphoric continuously during her 10-14 day change in behavior. She recalls instances of being appropriately upset during that time.
—Dr. Cohen does not conceptually object to psychiatric labeling of her experiences. She believes that Dr. Paltrow's Adjustment Disorder diagnosis is in keeping with her view of her REACTION to the April experience.

CLARIFICATION OF RECOMMENDATIONS
I believe that Dr. Cohen should not work as a physician during any possible future occurrences similar to her April experience. Dr. Cohen disagrees with me.

I do recommend at least monthly appointments with a psychiatrist in the first year of Dr. Cohen's return to work.

These would provide some degree of objective monitoring for possible unrecognized affective changes. The relationship with a psychiatrist would also allow urgent access to psychiatric treatment, if that became necessary.

I do NOT agree that Dr. Cohen currently needs lithium or other mood stabilizing medication.

I do NOT see psychotherapy as CONTRAindicated. If Dr. Cohen chooses to be in therapy, I think a psychologist, psychiatrist, or other licensed mental health professional would be appropriate. An exploratory psychotherapy could give her support in emotionally integrating her experiences of this past year. (In my October 14 letter, I did not intend to imply that Dr. Cohen needed therapy in order to alter her view of her experiences.) I believe that "hypnotic regression" would be unwise for Dr. Cohen.

FINAL THOUGHTS
Although it was not my intention, this letter does appear to me to document some affective intensity on Dr. Cohen's part, at least around this psychiatric evaluation. However, I do not see her as showing evidence of an uncontrolled mood disorder. Although I did not meet her before her experience, I see her intensity and detail orientation as parts of her personality, possibly exacerbated by her current professional stress. This view is supported by Dr. Bice's March and April therapy notes about her (not documenting any persisting personality change) and by her July 1998 screening psychological testing.

Sincerely,
Linda Thompson, MD

The problem I had with all of this was the implication that an experience of expanded consciousness could or should be classified by a system that identified only "disordered" or otherwise problematic state of mind. No official psychiatric perspectives considered expanded states of consciousness to be a normal part of our developmental evolution. Nor was there a place within the system for non-ordinary states of mind that were non-

Chapter 14: Four Moe Opinions

dysfunctional, minimally or temporarily dysfunctional in our "normal" development (such as adolescence), or hyperfunctional. And it seemed that those who had never experienced non-ordinary consciousness could not be enticed to take seriously the literature and objective research that supported the validity and value of such states of being.

10-21

...I sit outside, too noisy, move inside, walk through the garden, pick zucchini, putter around with this and that and find a day spent with little to show for itself. It's so discouraging.

I feel so lonely, adrift in a sea of disbelief and confrontation.

Invalidation is painful. Especially when the self is seeking to know the Self. Perhaps this is why we've developed as a society to not value our selves, but rather to value the opinions of others, of professionals, instead. It is not as painful to have things outside of ourselves discredited.

Someday we will all know. The outside, the inside, is all a part of who we are, all a part of the same thing.

October 23

Autumn. Let there be no more falls, only gentle descents.

The walnut tree leaves are golden. It matches the little maple in front of the basement window, which, too, is gold, only it has a touch of orange.

Outside my office window I can see our dahlias

Ghostwoman

still in full bloom, defying the cool weather. They'll be lovely until frost as long as I keep the spent, mushy, blossoms snipped off. The neighbor's pampas grass is silver and regal. Our pineapple sage, full of brilliant crimson plumes, and the other hummingbird perennial, the honey scented blue wispy thing, whatever it's called, is still full of blossoms. I think the hummingbirds have flown south for the winter, I haven't seen them for days. It was just last week that they were serenading each other around the sage, taking rests from their helicopter flight patterns in the lilac tree....

    My Friday is a mellow one. Frank practices piano and I have time to write. Mondeau desires someone to play ball with her. She asks with yips to go out and come in, and go out, and come in. I am too accommodating today, but she's such a love.

    I wonder what will be when my license is reinstated. This gentle existence feels meaningful today, despite my lack of productivity. Doesn't always feel this way. My prior existence felt too intense for me to think about the meaning of anything, and to continue as it was. It was devouring me.

    Meditation seems to help keep it all in perspective, though I overslept my morning meditation again. Still, remembering my breath reminds me about the passageways to other realities. No need to get too attached to this one. Love is all that is worth being attached to, and of that, there is plenty.

Chapter 14: Four Moe Opinions

I had not heard from Dr. Westman since I had seen him the previous month, and I placed a call to him to find out whether he had spoken with anyone on the Board as he had told me he would during my appointment with him. Expecting an assessment that did not portray my experience in pathological light, I wanted to make sure his opinion was on the record.

He returned my call to tell me that he had spoken with the Board, and would be sending them a written report within the next couple of days. I commented that they had a requirement that all documents needed to be in their hands by ten days before they met, and I was unsure if that meant ten working days. He reassured me that he had cleared this with the Board and that they would accept his report.

"Oh, and could you tell me what your final impression of my experience was?" I asked before hanging up the phone.

"I believe you had a single manic episode."

I was speechless.

David T. Bice Ph.D., P.C.
Clinical Psychologist

Oregon Board of Medical Examiners
620 Crown Plaza
1500 SW First Ave.
Portland Oregon 97201

Re: Dr. Harriet Cohen

To whom it may concern:

I have been asked to provide a summary of my findings as a result of my work with Dr. Cohen.
I have never seen Dr. Cohen display, nor report to me, a pattern of symptoms, which suggested the diagnosis of bipolar disorder.
She has reported a brief period of dissociation, which is not inconsistent with patterns of delayed or complicated grief.

Ghostwoman

As she is now, and I believe, will continue to address these grief issues, her emotional health has significantly improved. I would expect continued improvement with no further intrusions of dissociation.

She has made arrangements with me to follow up on a monthly basis as long as is necessary.

At this point it is my impression that she is at least as psychologically healthy and competent as she was prior to the emergence and onset of this experience/episode.

Sincerely
D.T. Bice Ph.D.

"... brief period of dissociation..." what a shame to have to label the only non-dissociated time of my life by its very opposite.

Chapter 15
The Hearing

The kids and I joined neighbors for their annual pumpkin carving contest. It was our first year to attend, and we'd excitedly gotten a number of very large pumpkins to carve while we met the people who lived all around us. Between the large lots and the tall hedges and fences, it was difficult to get to know each other. I liked feeling part of a neighborhood again. We were headed to the home of the family directly behind us, so I couldn't drive in good conscience, yet I could barely lift the pumpkins one at a time.

Iyra grabbed the wheelbarrow, and Jade the old rusty red wagon, and we loaded up our pumpkins and began lugging them around our yard, up our little hill and out our back gate. It was a clear fall day and the sun beat down on us as we tugged and pushed our wagons across the barely bridged ditch that separated our yards, then up the hill of another neighbor's backyard. Too bad we didn't have the downhill journey on the way there, and the uphill journey on the way back when the pumpkins had been emptied of their insides, carved, and were substantially lighter.

Iyra and Jade were shy about being around new people. Iyra was so reserved that she even passed her pumpkin over to me to do the carving. She had picked out the roundest, fattest, thickest pumpkin that she could find. Tables were set out on the front yard of the home and we all stood shoulder-to-shoulder with our elbows deep in pumpkin guts. I carved a peaceful cat-eyed Buddha face with a spiritual eye in the middle of a triangle in her forehead. Won first prize!

That evening I accompanied Paula to a drumming event hosted by the owner of one of the local Native American drum shops. The drum circle was led by an African man who had founded the World Federation for Spiritual Healing. We drummed, we danced, and he led us in various energy meditations before talking about the power of Love to heal. This was a message that I could not stop hearing. It was as if the Universe was making sure that despite the difficulties I was having professionally, I did not forget what the mystical experience was all about. It was feeding me vitamins of reassurance as my hearing with the Board drew near.

The following weekend, only days before my hearing, I received another boost of support at a regional Holistic Medical Association conference. I'd received a brochure in the mail that told me about the organization and their upcoming meeting at the coast. Although it was a bulk mailing, it felt like a personal invitation. This was the local chapter of a twenty-five-year-old medical organization, whose most fundamental precept is that Love Heals.

I spent three days in a two story-hotel complex nestled in a coastal forest by the ocean. The workshops on nonstandard healing modalities were interesting, but the treasure of the conference was fellow practitioners who'd had unusual personal experiences of their own. Their practices reflected their brilliant scientific minds, deeply caring hearts, and belief that the spiritual aspect of our

Chapter 15: The Hearing

world impacts our health profoundly— personally and professionally. One of the internists, Debra, even led a workshop that included teaching a form of muscle energy testing, a variant of my thumb thing. She used it in her practice for patients interested in experimenting with flower essence therapy. I listened to the stories of a number of the physicians who'd had their own cases against the Board at one time or another. They were a courageous, loving, playful group of men and women, between twenty-eight and seventy-seven years of age, whose integrity and desire to provide the broadest range of healing opportunities for their patients took priority over fears of retribution by the governing medical establishment.

The last day of the conference, cold wind blew fiercely, as it often does at the coast. It kept me from lingering outdoors after the conference ended and I headed home, frequently turning off the road to watch the massive waves crashing against the volcanic shoreline. Sea foam swirled violently and blew off the crests of the waves in the wind. The waves exploded onto the rocky shore into thunder. Sea palms, those cute little seaweed forms that look like foot high palm trees, taught me what it meant to be grounded and resilient. They were blasted repeatedly against their volcanic moorings but stayed tightly bound to the lava, bouncing back wave after wave after wave.

The house was a mess! Why was it that whenever I left for a few days it looked like a cyclone had hit?!! Dishes in the living room, along with half-eaten pieces of candy and all sorts of candy wrappers. The pot with unpopped corn kernels and butter sat on the floor next to the sofa. Dirty socks and Halloween costumes littered the floor; sections of the sofa were overturned; all the cushions messed up; toys, books, all over the place; the kitchen full of dirty dishes; the counter tops all unwiped. And

Mondeau's half chewed sticks had left a trail of slivers all over the house.

I had grabbed the mail on my way in and found Dr. Westman's report. It was on par with Dr. Eugene's. I could not even read the whole thing; it made me furious just to hold it! I threw it down on the mess-covered dining room table with the rest of the mail.

"Why can't you guys clean up after yourselves!?" I roared to no one in particular. "Look at this place!"

I am not a little seaweed palm tree, I am only human. My evening meditation filled with tears. At the coast they were tears of love, but here I was, once again, filled with frustration and animosity.

Monday morning I stopped in to see Thomas, and gave him a copy of a letter I had written, hoping the Board could receive it before I met with them later that week. He thought the letter would be fine and assured me he'd get it to the Board that day.

October 28, 1998

Edmond Deutsch, M.D. Chair
Oregon Board of Medical Examiners
620 Crown Plaza
1500 SW First Avenue
Portland, OR 97201-5826

Dear Dr. Deutsch and the Oregon Board of Medical Examiners,

This letter clarifies my position on my experience this past spring, my series of evaluations, and my personal recommendations for the resolution of my case.

It is clear that the psychiatric diagnosis for my experience is controversial, as there has been a lack of consensus amongst the professionals in this field. I myself have understood this experience diagnostically in an evolving way. Most helpful for me in understanding this experience has been a book by Dennis Gersten, MD, a

Chapter 15: The Hearing

psychiatrist who has long studied spiritual experiences, and whose book, <u>Are you Getting Enlightened or Losing Your Mind?</u> offers definitions and distinctions that separate spiritual experiences, such as I experienced, from states of mental illness. This distinction is very important for two reasons. Prognosticly, Dr. Gersten explains the *positive* transformative nature of spiritual experiences (pp. 179-180), as opposed to the negative cycle of relapses and dysfunction that accompanies mental illness. Secondly, it has supported my own credibility (pp. 108-111, 188-190) from a psychiatric source, which was taken away by Dr. Eugene's limited ability to understand my experience as anything but "delusional." By defining my experience as an illness, it becomes identified as a disease state, as opposed to an experience of profound and lasting value, marking the beginning of a period of spiritual growth and awakening.

That said, I can appreciate your apprehension with this model, as these distinctions and understandings are not yet to be found in standard psychiatric literature. Conventional psychiatry has not sincerely honored the reality of spiritual experiences, and so has not valued the studies that differentiate these experiences from mental illness.

What is evident to me from this process of multiple evaluations is that I could be seen by many more psychiatrists without knowledge of spiritual experiences and receive some sort of a mood disorder diagnosis from all of them. This is the only choice they have; this is all they know. I could also be seen by psychiatrists who have knowledge and understanding of spiritual states, and receive a very different classification. Thus I acknowledge that the diagnosis of my experience was, and continues to be, subjective and a reflection of the experiences, beliefs, and fears of my evaluators.

To help resolve some of the subjectivity, I did consent to formal, objective testing. This did not uncover mental illness, but only identified personality traits that have become even more apparent through this ordeal:

1) The patient is naïve.
Having imagined that armed with books and articles by prominent psychiatrists in this field, I could effect the

nonspiritual mindset of psychiatric diagnosis, was, admittedly, very naïve of me.

2) "...*patient might have attempted to present an unrealistically favorable picture of her personal virtue and moral values.*"
This reminds me of the quote from Jesus' sermon on the mount, "Blessed are the pure in heart: for they shall see God...." To this end, perhaps those within the field of psychiatry might work a little harder on themselves. Personal virtue, integrity, love, and moral values are quite attainable, as are the spiritual experiences that frequently accompany them. Only by experiencing these firsthand, can psychiatry hope to evaluate such experiences out of wisdom, rather than from ignorance.

In conclusion, I accept your concerns and fears in dealing with the ambiguity of my case. To resolve my case I ask that:
1. My license be reinstated, as all my recent psychiatric evaluations, including the objective testing, attest to my lack of psychiatric impairment.
2. Acknowledgment is made that my medical decision making was never impaired.
3. No official diagnosis of this experience be settled on, as there has been no consensus amongst professionals in the psychiatric and psychological field. I would like to recommend that for the record, it be stated that, 'Dr. Cohen had a spiritual experience that was accompanied by changes in her mood, behavior, counseling strategies, and professional charting. Specific diagnosis from a psychiatric perspective remains controversial.'
4. If the Board feels it necessary for their own peace of mind, follow-up visits with a psychiatrist of my choosing be required for a maximum of six more months.
As I acknowledge your position of uncertainty regarding this situation, I would also recommend that should I someday return to a similar state of altered consciousness, I be reevaluated by a licensed psychiatrist of my choosing.

Lastly, I would like to apologize for the angry tone of my and my lawyer's letter to you. It was inspired by what I perceived, and still perceive, as violations of my rights and invasions of my privacy. This, however, is a separate issue

Chapter 15: The Hearing

that perhaps we could discuss, so hopefully some changes can be made in your procedures that will be less hurtful and alienating to the physicians under your review.

Sincerely,
Harriet Cohen, MD

I skimmed through Dr. Grof's books that afternoon, soothed by his words.

"Many of the states that psychiatry considers to be manifestations of mental diseases of unknown origin are actually expressions of a self-healing process in the psyche and in the body..." And later in his book, "Because of the vast available literature on unitive experiences, we have not included an essay on this subject in the present work. We highly recommend Maslow's work for further study."

Vast available literature on unitive experiences.

I marked that passage and page. Might come in handy.

Each page I read about the healing potential and POSITIVE value of experiences such as mine made me a little more confident, erasing the opinions that had invalidated me. I read a couple dozen pages before it was time to fix dinner and get the kids to bed.

I'd arranged to meet Thomas in his office the morning of the hearing, and from there we would walk to the Oregon Board of Medical Examiners office, only a few blocks away.

"Good morning! How are you holding up?" Thomas asked congenially.

"Pretty good, all things considered. I stopped off at a new doctor's office yesterday and she fixed me up with some flower essences for courage. They seem to be working. I'm feeling more interested in this hearing than worried about it." I smiled.

The sky was clear and fresh. Some of the trees were

still changing color, but most had lost their leaves, which carpeted the sidewalks, crunching under our feet.

We passed my car on our way, and I stopped to feed my parking meter. As I ratcheted in my quarters, Thomas bent over to pick up a penny he saw lying on the sidewalk. "This is a good sign," he said. "I was in Hawaii a few years back. I'd taken myself there to try and pull my life together after my first wife asked me for a divorce. It hit me like a sledge hammer, totally out of the blue. So there I was in Hawaii, sitting quietly one day, meditating by a rock, and when I opened my eyes, there was a penny in front of me that I hadn't seen before. I picked it up and as I looked at it, the words **'In God We Trust'** just jumped out at me."

In God we trust. Always there, always looking out for us, and always with our long-term best interests in mind. Hard to believe sometimes. I guess that's why we need all the reminders.

We arrived ten minutes early and sat down in the small waiting room. Two other men were already seated on the other leg of the "L"-shaped seating arrangement. On the end table next to me I noticed one of the magazines had a cover article about alternative healing modalities of native cultures. Thomas sat next to me on the other side and filled me in a bit more on what the room we'd be going into would look like. He had already prepared me for what to expect. He didn't think the Board was at all interested in my meditative experience, but rather that they just wanted to be sure that I was not in any way a threat to patients, and that I was of sound mind. He'd counseled me to not say anything more than what was asked of me. He would nudge my arm if I started talking too much.

I expected to be asked questions, and I expected to answer them honestly and succinctly. I had brought two of my books along, just in case the opportunity arose to share psychiatric support for my perspective on my case.

Chapter 15: The Hearing

I did begin to worry a bit because the Board was running late. We learned from another man in the waiting room that the physician being grilled before me was a mess, in tears, and the process was taking longer than usual. I was not concerned about my hearing but about my parking meter. Thomas could only laugh. Here he was, sitting next to me at $175.00 an hour and I was worried about a potential twelve-dollar parking ticket. He gave me some change for the meter and I took a little stroll to my car.

The sun wrapped its tentacles of warmth around me. I passed a number of cars whose meters were just about to run out or already had. The meter maid was on the other side of the street writing tickets, so I fed the empty and near empty meters along my way, then filled up my own before heading back.

Swish, swish went the leaves beneath my shoes. The fallen leaves caught my attention and I saw a curious yellow and green maple leaf in a sea of red and brown oak. I looked up and around but couldn't see the tree from which this maple leaf had fallen. Yellow and green, the colors of my aura, according to another wholeness center friend. I picked it up for good luck, smiled at the day, and disappeared back into the building.

Our wait continued. Bored, I struck up a conversation with the other two people in the waiting room. Actually, I spoke mainly with one of them. The other, holding a movie camera, was the silent type with whom little eye contact could be made.

The man I spoke to was a reporter doing a story on the Oregon Board of Medical Examiners for a local news network. His question was whether or not the Board was serving its constituents well, the constituents being the taxpayers, who should know if a particular physician has complaints lodged against him or her. The reporter had already sat through a number of hearings and was, in fact, the one who told us about the unfortunate doctor who was currently being dissected by the Board.

Thomas and I both perked up. Without revealing too much about our case, we did our best to alert the reporter to the other side of the problem with the Board: their lack of due process and the problem of discriminating against practitioners who integrated complementary medicine into their practices. Thomas handed the reporter his card.

Finally, an hour after my appointed time, I was called into the hearing room. It was very large, with about ten boardroom tables set in a semicircle around the perimeter of the far half of the room. Conservative-looking men in suits and ties sat behind them facing a lonely table in the center of the room with two chairs, one for me and one for Thomas. I was glad he had accompanied me.

We sat facing most of the tables, but two of them continued down the side of the room, beyond my field of vision. Additionally, there were chairs lined up behind us for observers of one sort or another, including the reporters and the investigators who had come up to my home.

So began the inquisition.

Contrary to Thomas's expectations, they began by asking me to tell them in my own words what I experienced that day while meditating. This I was most happy to do, as I always receive a peculiar feeling of joy when talking about the experience of Oneness and Absolute Love.

Then one after another, the IC members fired a barrage of questions at me. I remained calm and clear with my answers, even with those questions that seemed meant to unnerve me.

"Tell me, Dr. Cohen, are you familiar with denial?" one of the members asked as he leaned back in his armchair looking down at me over the tops of his glasses. "And could you tell me how a patient in denial might present?"

I answered him calmly. "There could be a number of presentations starting with projection. A patient who can't

Chapter 15: The Hearing

see something about themselves might project it onto someone else. They also might present with multiple somatic complaints for which no identifiable etiology can be found."

This particular member kept doing his best to corner me into admitting whatever wrongdoing he could conceive of. He zeroed in on my charting omissions, which I admitted were not as good as they could have been. His wording was something like, "So, you admit that your charting was beneath the standard of practice..."

I was handed copies of some of my chart notes and asked to read them aloud. Included were notes about a three-hundred pound patient who had come in with shoulder complaints. I was struck with the beauty of her face that day, and charted it. I read the record aloud.

"And do you think that what you wrote is sufficient? A patient comes in with complaints of shoulder pain and there is no examination of the patient?"

"You've given me a chart note to read out of context from the rest of the chart. This was a chronic problem, and it is quite possible that there is a documented exam of the patient on the visit before. However, it is quite possible that there is only a limited exam anywhere in the chart because I am not very good at doing orthopedic exams of shoulders in heavy set patients. The patient had an appointment with the orthopedist the following week, so I chose to use our time to deal with some of her self-esteem issues."

I remember one more specific period of questioning. It was when it was time to be questioned by the psychiatric consultant for the Board. He was seated somewhat behind me and the microphone was directly in front of me. I was trying to look at this man and answer his questions when I was told to please speak into the microphone, requiring a very awkward craning of my neck. "I'm going to need a chiropractor when I'm done here," I timidly quipped. A few chuckles emerged from the audience before I quickly added, "I hope I'm allowed to say that in here." More laughter, my own included, and it took me a moment to compose myself.

As I spoke my case for spiritual experiences being distinct from mental illness, I was almost able to reference my books. "I've brought them with me if you'd like to see them," I said. Heads nodded and I pulled them out. Unfortunately, the opportunity did not arise for me to share more than the titles and the authors. They wanted to ask *me* the questions; they did not care to hear the opinions of the professionals in my books who had spent lifetimes studying this subject.

The psychiatrist for the Board at one point inferred that I didn't think that patients with mental illness needed to be treated with medications. "No," I corrected him, "This is one of the distinctions between spiritual experiences and mental illness. Patients suffering from mental illness often needed, and were helped by medications in order to function; whereas patients having spiritual experiences generally need only guidance and emotional support while their symptoms abate spontaneously."

After it was all over, the woman who had led me into the room offered to lead me out another door, to avoid the reporters. I had nothing to hide and so politely declined, leaving through the same door I had entered. Once in the foyer, I took a deep breath.

"You did great!" said Thomas. "I had nothing to do but listen!"

Now all there was to do, once again, was to wait.

That afternoon, Frank called from work. When I heard his voice I thought that he was concerned about how things had gone with the Board, and interested in how I was doing.

"Harriet, could you check on the phone number for the Tibetan medicine conference I'm going to? I need to

Chapter 15: The Hearing

double-check my reservations."

Before he hung up, I asked if he wanted to know how things went? It seemed by his pause that my question had jogged his memory about something I had going on that day. Fine, I answered, trying very hard to maintain a humored mindset about my husband's absentmindedness about my circumstances; about me.

November 7

Saturday morning. Shabbat.

I was too tired last night to attend the musical happening at the Wholeness center. Even Rochelle's personal invitation, and hearing about other friends who would be there wasn't enough to move me. I was exhausted and needed to sleep.

So it was that at 8 pm I kicked off my boots and landed in bed, fully clothed with even my coat still on. Frank was off in D.C. at the Tibetan medicine conference, so I'd asked the kids to clean up the dishes from dinner and to put themselves to bed. I hadn't yet looked to see how much they accomplished.

At 10 p.m. Iyra tearfully woke me up, realizing that she'd lost her swim-meet suit. With a meet in the morning, no swim suit, and Shabbat closing the center for the day, even her practice suit would not available.

I rooted around the house with half-open eyes, sadly unable to help her find it. I knew I'd seen it somewhere, but where??? Instead, I found an old leotard that would probably work as a back up, so I put her to bed with the promise that if they sold

Ghostwoman

suits at the meet, which they often did, that I would get her a new one.

    Iyra decided she wanted to sleep in my bed with me. Her alarm didn't work and she wanted to be by one since she needed to wake up early. Whatever the reason, it was nice to have her so near.

> I love to watch the sun set.
> Even when, on days like today,
> My eyelids grow heavy and my body weary.
> I watch the golden globe
> settle into gray pillows for the night.
> The canvas ever changing,
> One most beautiful painting
> Absorbing into the next.
> Softer glows the glow
> Sinking into thicker haze,
> and clouds, and gray,
> until it showers pinks and oranges,
> purples and gold
> across the sky
> while I
> fight sleep
> to keep
> the priceless sky
> before my eyes.

    Frank returned from his conference in D.C. in a much calmer and happier state of mind than I had known him to be in a long time. There was much that I had wanted to tell him, share with him, teach and learn with him from

Chapter 15: The Hearing

my books and my mystical experience. But when I'd tried, it had not gone well. He hadn't seemed open or interested in hearing about these things from me. And I was afraid to share too much, as I had all I could bear with having these truths, *my truths,* rejected by my medical community, and perhaps my Rabbi as well (though I did not have the courage to ask him any more about this directly). I knew I could not handle confrontation from Frank, too.

But he had heard from his holiness the Dali Lama and his Llama entourage.

"It was their clarity that helped me to understand the connection between emotions and physical health," he said, looking peacefully into my eyes with love.

How clear his eyes shined as he told me about the conference. His strong body even seemed to be softer and more animated than usual as he described the Tibetan notion of afflictive emotions. And he seemed to be simply describing it. I didn't get the sense that he was talking down to me, as I often did when he wanted to tell me about something. He was just enjoying sharing the knowledge he had learned, knowledge that somehow had helped awaken something inside him.

The kids and I gathered in the living room around the old coffee table when Frank brought out the little gifts he'd bought for us. I sat on the edge of the sofa while the rest of my family kneeled and sat on the floor.

"Hand made Tibetan incense," Frank said, unwrapping bundle after bundle of various shaped sticks. Then he opened a package containing four small, shimmering, woven bags about the size of the palm of my childrens' hands. Each had a woven rope attached to it so that they could be worn around the neck. "There's a Sanskrit blessing inside, and they've been blessed by the Dali Lama. They're supposed to bring protection."

I felt a warm joy fill me as I thought about the tradition in Judaism to wear a *Mezuzah* around the neck, as well as to attach them to the door posts of our homes. These, too, were small, ornate, containers. But they were made of wood, metal, or ceramic, and enclosed were Hebrew verses from the Torah:

HEAR O ISRAEL: THE LORD OUR GOD, THE LORD IS ONE.

And thou shalt love the Lord thy God with all thy heart, and with all thy soul, and with all thy might. And these words, which I command thee this day, shall be upon thy heart; and thou shalt teach them diligently unto thy children, and shalt talk of them when thou sittest in thy house, and when thou walkest by the way, and when thou liest down, and when thou risest up...

The last thing that Frank brought out was a package filled with multicolored grains of sand. "The monks were creating this intricate sand art design, and at the end of the conference, they swept all the sand together and passed out the sand to whoever wanted some. It's supposed to bring good luck."

It had already done that, I thought to myself as I went off to get the perfect glass container. It had brought peace to Frank.

11-11-98

...I feel myself shifting from my county practice into some sort of holistic program development, education, and research. On my own? Yikes!!

How quickly? When to begin? By the need, yesterday. By the inertia of motherhood— God only knows. My family is important to me. I'm grateful that my thumbs agree there is not such a hurry that I must step further away from my mothering

Chapter 15: The Hearing

work than I already have.

They seem to be doing well with my new direction in life and my need for time to read and write. They support me. Believe in me and in what I am doing.

What AM I doing?

11-14-98

Hiking with myself. Our family hike. The kids weren't interested, only wanted to stay home and play computer games. I brought along my camera instead. A very pleasant afternoon filled with awareness of the electric beauty of a lovely stretch of the Pacific Crest trail. An evergreen forest with views of a few hills that still had some trees. Patches of lichen growing wild designs onto the rocks. A little creek now and then to stone-step over. Patches of lingering snow. I paused as I pleased, and enjoyed the quiet.

My hike behind me, I enjoyed the drive home, listening to tapes of my choice for a change. A series of talks by Thich Nhat Hanh.

"Our actions are our only true belongings... Love is made of understanding. Understanding comes from looking deeply...

"Love is action. The symbol of love is a hand...."

These Buddhist teachings are like Jewish teachings. The importance of action is central to Judaism.

I remember the esoteric Jewish video of a small metal sculpture that fit inside the palm of a hand.

The shadows created by this sculpture when a light was shined upon it created the whole Hebrew alphabet. A Christian Wholeness Center friend had shared that video with me. Thanks again, Blanche!

"The goal of love is to bring joy and transform suffering....

"Love has the power to heal. Love is the power to heal."

I finished his tape on love and switched to one on mindfulness. There he spoke about the importance of space: to not be so project-oriented that we suck up all the space and forget who we are. I know what he's talking about. My mind, sometimes, a flood of projects. My book. My article. Creating/bringing a holistic health model to the county health department—if they would have it. Creating a holistic healing coalition? Involving myself in the needs of my community. Continuing to work with our various schools for the kids.

And where will this time come from to do all of these things?

Betsy had been holding my job open for me, and after receiving Dr. Paltrow's report, had told me to let her know if there was anything she could do to help move things along. We arranged to meet her over breakfast.

I was the first to arrive at the little French cafe she recommended. It was halfway between my home and her office, and on this midmorning weekday only one other table was occupied. The room was otherwise filled with the smell of fresh coffee, frying eggs, sautéed vegetables and melted cheese.

Chapter 15: The Hearing

I sat down and anxiously waited. My heart was thumping loudly and my hands were a little moist and shaky. It was curious to me that I had not felt so nervous in front of the Investigative Committee. But they were not my boss, and I was firm in my convictions about what I was discussing with them, as opposed to my uncertainty about what I wanted to say to Betsy. I'd been thinking a lot, meditating, talking to God with my thumbs, and talking to friends. I wanted to work more with the connection between spirituality and health but did not quite know in what way I would do this. I was still wondering about it all when Betsy walked in.

"It's good to see you," she said with a warm smile. "You look great."

"Thanks, so do you." She always looked so together with her neat hair and not too conservative clothes. "How are things at the county?"

"Busy as usual," she answered. Then she told me some of the various politics I had missed during my absence.

"But what's going on with you? How's your leg?"

"Oh, it's coming along. I've been taking advantage of my time off and learning yoga. That's done wonders for my leg. It still hurts if I carry anything, and I can't walk too far without feeling some pain, but it's getting better."

"What was the deal with the person who hit you?" Betsy asked.

"Who knows," I answered. "She's claiming she had a seizure."

"That would explain it."

"Not exactly. Not to me, anyway. Some of the details just don't make sense. But I've got a lawyer dealing with that. I had to file a lawsuit to try and get any compensation. Under Oregon law a seizure is an act of God, so she's not considered to be negligent and has no legal responsibility for any of the consequences of the accident. And if one lawsuit wasn't enough, we've filed two. The second one is against the property owners. My accident was the twelfth time a car had crashed through one of the storefronts and they still hadn't put up any barriers."

"You're kidding!" said Betsy incredulously.

"Wish I was. Dealing with lawyers isn't exactly my favorite thing in the world, and now I've got two of them. But they're both great people."

Betsy shifted in her chair. "How are things going with the Board? What's the status with your license?"

"I'm waiting," I answered. "I finally had my interview on the fifth, and now I'm waiting to hear back from the Investigative Committee to see what's going to happen next.

"How did the hearing go?"

"It wasn't bad. It actually felt pretty good. My lawyer thought things went well, too. Even the reporters who were there thought I spoke up for myself well."

"There were reporters?" Betsy scrunched up one side of her face a bit.

"Yup. They were there doing some kind of story about the Board, and we were waiting together in the waiting room for about an hour before my hearing. I even got on the camera on my way out."

"You don't want to get involved with the media," she warned. Then she continued, "Do you have any idea how long it'll be before you hear from the Board?"

"I don't. Thomas thinks it shouldn't be too long. But that's just the Investigative Committee. Then they'll have to give their recommendations to the Board for their final approval, or absolution, or whatever it is that they do. One of the papers I received stated it would take three to four weeks. I'm not sure if that's after the hearing or after the Board gives their final O.K."

"It must be stressful to be waiting like this," Betsy said.

"It hasn't been too bad. I started writing a book about

Chapter 15: The Hearing

the whole thing, so that keeps me busy."

"I'll bet that's therapeutic."

I felt myself bristle a bit, misinterpreting her words to mean that the writing was ONLY of therapeutic value, when I felt the issues to be important and global ones. "I've also appreciated the time I've had to read more about the connection between meditation and healing. There's a lot that's been researched on this subject." I had brought Betsy a book on the subject by Herbert Benson M.D. shortly after I'd been placed on leave. That was when I was still going to meetings, thinking the leave would be over in days, or at the most, a couple of weeks.

"I'm envious about your time to read," she said between forkfuls of breakfast.

"It's amazing stuff!" I added exuberantly, my love for this field of medicine becoming somewhat uncontainable. Then I felt my nervousness heat up again. It was time to bring up what I'd most wanted, but was most afraid to talk about.

"In fact, I'm discovering it's so beneficial that I want to figure out how to teach it, how to reach more patients and reach them most effectively. Maybe even do some sort of study on the benefit of teaching meditation to county clients. There's not enough time to do everything in the short visits we have with patients. Maybe I could lead some sort of a group."

"There's no money for you to do that," she answered matter-of-factly. "We do have some groups starting up, but they won't be taught by physicians. We'll use the psych Nurse Practitioners and probably the social workers."

I was hoping to somehow maintain my connection with the county and continue to work for them, perhaps funded by a grant of some sort. But the quiet reality that I had been trying to ignore, that I would need to resign from my position in order to pursue mindbody medicine, was becoming more and more clear.

"Your patients haven't had a consistent provider for over a year and a half now," Betsy reminded me.

I clicked off the list in my head. First my four-and-a-half-month sabbatical... back three months before I was off again for a two-week vacation. Back a month, then the accident. Off two months after the accident. Back for three months, then this.

"Recently we've hired an on-call physician to see some of your patients. She's been working out really well, but she's looking for a permanent job. If you're thinking of doing something different when this is all over, I'd like to know as soon as possible so that I can offer your position to her before she gets a position somewhere else."

I felt a little stunned at the abruptness of her request. I suspect that the ghostwoman came back to share my breakfast at that moment and protect me from my feelings. I had worked for the county for twelve and a half years; had postponed my much-needed time off when other providers left on short notice; had cared about my patients and cared about the health department; had worked beyond my paid hours covering patients for other physicians who had abruptly left the county.

The ghostwoman thought, 'We did have the patients to think about. It was hard to get replacement physicians when we needed them. What about my overworked colleagues?'

What about me?

I didn't ask that last question right away. I didn't ask that question for two years. And then, not until a writer giving me feedback on my story, asked how did I FEEL?

"How did you feel when your boss was thinking about everyone but you? How long did you work there? How many times had you covered for other physicians? How did it feel to be so dispensable?"

That was when I felt it: the vibration, the anger, the surge of energy from my feet through my body, through the tips of my fingers; all those things that I can't feel

Chapter 15: The Hearing

when I'm looking into the face of another human being. These sensations began filling me there in my friend's dining room, and they continued to ignite me with an energy of ferocity all my way home.

The sadness and anger we feel when we are not valued.

Chapter 16
First Response

I was on my own. Yet, I reminded myself I was never on my own; God was always working with me and through me. I let go of my worries about being a one-income family in this rapidly changing world where businesses collapse and jobs end abruptly. But habits die hard, and like a yo-yo my worries kept returning. I breathed fully. I meditated. And I sent my fears on their way again. Maybe someday this string would break. Someday I would live in the mind of surrender and trust, and could just be. Someday, fear would be a story I told my children about my past. Maybe someday.

Monday, November 23rd, I received correspondence from Thomas with the IC's official response to my hearing:

Dear Harriet:

Enclosed please find a copy of the letter from Mr. Herman of November 18 with the enclosed proposed Corrective Action Order, together with the packet of information regarding reactivation of your license.

Chapter 16: First Response

I believe there are some major problems with the proposed Order and want to discuss my views with you after you have had a chance to review it and "digest" it.

I have not retained a copy of the information packet, nor have I spent any time reviewing that.

Very truly yours,
Thomas E. McDermott

BEFORE THE
BOARD OF MEDICAL EXAMINERS
STATE OF OREGON

In the Matter of
Harriet Cohen, M.D.,   CORRECTIVE ACTION ORDER
License No. MD54321

1.

The Board of Medical Examiners (Board) is the state agency responsible for licensing, regulating and disciplining certain health care providers in the State of Oregon. Harriet Cohen, M.D. (Licensee) is a licensed physician in the state of Oregon.

2.

On or about April 1, 1998, the staff of the Multnomah County Health Department observed a significant change in the behavior of the Licensee. Following an audit of clinical charts for patients treated by the Licensee in the spring of 1998, Licensee was placed on administrative leave from the County Health Department. A psychiatrist subsequently evaluated Licensee, and diagnosed her as having a bipolar disorder. The Board, having been informed of Licensee's condition, had concerns about Licensee's ability to safely and competently practice medicine. In response to the Board's concern, the Licensee voluntarily withdrew from the practice of medicine pending the Board's review. At the Board's request, Licensee was subsequently evaluated by a psychiatrist selected by the Board, who assessed Licensee as having a mood disorder, and that she is now psychiatrically able to practice medicine.

3.

In regard to the above referenced matter, Licensee neither admits nor denies a violation of the Medical

Ghostwoman

Practices Act. For the purposes of resolving this investigation, Licensee and the Board agree to close this investigation contingent upon Licensee satisfying the following conditions:

3.1 Within three (3) business days of receipt of this order in a fully executed form, Licensee shall give written notice of the existence of this order, with a copy of the Order attached, to the Medical Director of Multnomah County Health Department, as well as the chief administrator of each business, hospital, card facility, or other institution in which Licensee has privileges or is employed or practices. Licensee shall also send a copy of this Order to any other entity with whom Licensee proposes to associate before practicing under the auspices of that entity. Licensee shall cause the Medical Director and such chief administrator(s) to report in writing to the Board by the last day of the month prior to each quarterly Board meeting. The report shall describe Licensee's compliance with the terms of this Order and comment on Licensee's ability to safely practice medicine, to the best of the reporters knowledge and judgment.

3.2 Licensee shall maintain a physician/patient relationship with a psychiatrist approved by the Board's Investigative Committee, who shall submit quarterly reports to the Board regarding Licensee's status and ability to safely and competently practice medicine.

3.3 Licensee is currently employed by the Multnomah County Health Department. In the event Licensee intends to change her place of employment to practice medicine, she must notify the Board's Investigative Committee at least thirty (30) days in advance of changing her employment.

4.

Evidence of violation of the terms of this agreement shall be grounds for discipline pursuant to ORS 677.190.

5.

Licensee agrees and understands that by entering into this Corrective Action Order, she waives her right to a contested case hearing or appeal therefrom.

IT IS SO STIPULATED this _____ day of _____, 1998.
     HARRIET Cohen, M.D.
IT IS SO ORDERED this _____ day of _____, 1998.
     BOARD OF MEDICAL EXAMINERS

Chapter 16: First Response

State of Oregon

J. Brice Walters, Jr., M.D.
Chairman of the Board

I found it incredible that the Board had crafted such a document, complete with the opinions of the psychiatrists they concurred with, but totally ignoring the dissenting opinions of other specialists as well as the testing that I had done. I also felt their statement that I "neither admit or deny a violation of the Medical Practices Act" implied that there was some problem in this regard. I denied this vehemently! And I could not understand why I needed to agree to show this document to all future employers.

Having resigned from my job, I was no longer in a hurry to get things wrapped up. More important to me, was my desire for the IC and the Board to acknowledge the differences between spiritual experiences and mental illness. I felt like the defender of something very holy. It was my job to vindicate the mystical experience, if not in the hearts and minds of those who judged me, at least legally and in writing.

"How can they create such a biased document?" I asked Thomas.

"They can do whatever they want. But we don't have to sign it."

I pointed out the specific problems that I had with the order, and Thomas concurred. We also agreed that it was totally unreasonable for them to set limitations on me indefinitely.

"What do we do now?" I asked.

"I'll write a letter clarifying our position, then send it to you to review before sending it to the Board."

Frank picked up my journal one day and called my writing about him poison.

"I don't just write bad stuff about you, I write whatever's going on on the days I have time to write.

"What did I write that made you so angry?"

"I'm not angry."

His voice was calm but his eyes flared. "Frank, You blame me for Mondeau possibly getting pregnant, as if I was irresponsible and let her out. We don't even know if she's pregnant! Maybe she has swollen nipples for some other reason.

"Yet my license has been suspended for seven months, I'm going through this ordeal with the Board, and you never ask me how things are going. I need to feel like you care about me, not just the dog. Ask me how I feel sometimes."

"I know how you feel and I know what you want. I don't give it to you so you can learn how to take care of yourself."

It had been barely tolerable to think that he never asked because he didn't know any better. But to hear him say he thought he knew what I wanted from our relationship and consciously withheld it hurt so deeply that my longing for intimacy became longing for separation.

"Our conversations are always so superficial and meaningless," he said.

"I agree."

But we couldn't seem to move any further. We couldn't talk about the hard stuff without feeling hurt and criticized, so we didn't. Instead, I expressed my frustrations in my journal. Poison.

Where to go from there? To clean out the basement for the friend who needed a place to live and was about to move in with us.

Wed. 25th 2:07 am

Frank reached out for me tonight and I returned his touch. I do not want to be angry with him. I thought of our last argument, what was it all about anyway? Will we ever figure out what we each need to not feel so hurt by the other during the next disagreement?

    I do not know what he needs, and he doesn't tell me. I know what I need. I need to be accepted, all of me. And if I'm enraged or angry, I need someone to simply say, 'You seem so angry, or unhappy, is there anything I can do to help?' I need him to listen. Just listen. Without judgment, without criticism, and without telling me what I need to do to "fix" myself. What works for him does not necessarily work for me. Just listening with empathy would help so much to lessen my anger or my sadness.

On December 4th, Thomas received a letter from the Board informing us about a conference call with the full Board on December 3rd. It was the first time we'd been notified of that date and we had not gotten our response back to the Board yet, due to the long Thanksgiving weekend.

Dear Mr. McDermott:

It is my understanding that you have some concerns with the Board's proposed Corrective Action Order for Dr. Cohen's signature. Please be advised that it is the Board's intention to facilitate Dr. Cohen's expedient return to her practice of medicine. To that end, the Board drafted the Corrective Action Order which is non-reportable and sets forth those terms and conditions that Dr. Cohen told the Investigative Committee of the Board she would be willing to comply with. I was hoping to have it approved at the full Board conference call on December 3rd, so that Dr. Cohen could return to practice.

It is the Board's understanding that you have concerns about the indefinite time period during which the order is in

Ghostwoman

effect. The Board is willing to review the corrective action order after one year at Dr. Cohen's request. At that review the Board will determine if further reports confirming Dr. Cohen's ability to safely practice medicine are necessary.

We would like your client's response to this clarification as soon as possible so that we can proceed as expeditiously as possible.

Thank you for your attention to this matter.

Very truly yours,
Catherine Harvey, JD
Executive Director

Thomas fired back our frustrations:

Dear Ms. Harvey:

    I have your letter of December 4, 1998, concerning my client, Dr. Cohen. First, in view of the many delays and other procedural "run-arounds" documented in the file, I find your comments regarding the Board's alleged intent to "facilitate Dr. Cohen's expedient return to her practice of medicine" and your desire to proceed "as expeditiously as possible" to be transparently self serving. For example, Mr. Herman's letter of November 18th, 1998, which enclosed the proposed Corrective Action Order fails to make any mention of a December 3 Board conference call or to otherwise alert me to the desirability of responding by a certain date. Indeed, a phone call or a fax (as opposed to a letter sent by surface mail) would have allowed Dr. Cohen and I to move more quickly in responding.

    Second, the allegation that the proposed Corrective Action Order simply sets forth terms and conditions that "Dr. Cohen told the Investigative Committee of the Board she would be willing to comply with" is false. I invite you to transcribe the tape-recorded comments from Dr. Cohen at the Investigative Committee interview to confirm what Dr. Cohen actually said. While Dr. Cohen was willing to consider further monitoring by a psychiatrist acceptable to the Board

Chapter 16: First Response

and herself, there was never any suggestion that the time period would be indefinite. More importantly, she was never asked, nor did she agree, to limit her ability to seek new or different employment or to require her supervisors or employers to report quarterly to the Board.

For your information, I am enclosing a copy of my letter to Dr. Walters which Dr. Cohen requests the immediate scheduling of a contested case hearing although she remains open to a reasonable compromise. I continue to be dismayed by the Board's heavy-handed treatment of this very fine physician who has devoted her career to caring for the indigent.

Very truly yours,
Thomas E. McDermott

The letter to Dr. Walters was our official response to the Corrective Action Order. In it we stated:

"... The Interim Stipulated Order provides in Paragraph 4 that the Board will investigate "in an expeditious manner" whether Dr. Cohen may safely return to the practice of medicine. The Board has apparently concluded its investigation but has failed to state its conclusion regarding Dr. Cohen's competence to return to practice. Instead, the Board has proposed a Corrective Action Order that:
—Misstates her clinical course of treatment and evaluation; (It is particularly offensive to Dr. Cohen that the Board included only the misdiagnosis of Dr. Eugene and the unspecified mood disorder finding of Dr. Thompson while ignoring the findings of Drs. Paltrow and Bice.)
—Interferes with her freedom of contract regarding employment as a physician;
—Requires her to "cause" supervising medical directors or administrators to report in writing to the Board at least four times a year; and
—Requires her to maintain a physician/patient relationship with a psychiatrist who is to report to the Board quarterly on her ability to safely and competently practice medicine.

Ghostwoman

Most incredibly, there is no stated time limit on these requirements. Theoretically, it would extend for the remainder of her professional career.

We are aware of no rationale for these proposed requirements, nor has the Board stated any. The psychiatrist selected by the Board for an independent evaluation, Dr. Thompson, concluded in her report of October 14, 1998 that Dr. Cohen had a spiritual experience and that she was "now psychiatrically able to practice medicine." As a precaution, however, Dr. Thompson suggested that Dr. Cohen be followed for one year "for periodic monitoring of her mood and for rapid access to treatment, if necessary."

Moreover, Dr. Paltrow, Dr. Cohen's treating psychiatrist, tested her extensively, found no evidence of a mood disorder and that she was competent to return to the practice of medicine with a good prognosis. Dr. Paltrow recommended that Dr. Cohen continue to see her psychologist, Dr. Bice, as needed.

In view of the Board's failure to comply with the terms of the Interim Stipulated Order (i.e., to expeditiously reach a conclusion regarding Dr. Cohen's ability to safely return to practice), she has no choice but to request a hearing. Alternatively Dr. Cohen is prepared to reach a reasonable compromise agreeing to quarterly psychiatric evaluations for one year. Based on the objective medical evidence, there is no reasonable basis to impair her ability to seek new or different employment or to continue psychiatric "monitoring" for more than one year. Please advise if the Board wishes to pursue such a compromise.

Very truly yours,
Thomas E. McDermott

* * * * *

At this same time my other legal adventure began to require some attention.

It had been over a year since the bakery accident. I'd been receiving regular correspondence about the case, but otherwise contact with Ted Goldstein, my lawyer was

Chapter 16: First Response

minimal. Depositions, scheduled and postponed three times, were finally taken on the tenth of December.

I met with Ted and Mary, his assistant, beforehand in Ted's office in one of the downtown towers. Ted sat behind his large desk and I sat in one of the two leather swivel chairs on the other side. Behind me, plate glass windows revealed a sweeping view of the city.

"Did you ever get the documents with her cell phone records?" I asked. I had seen Ted's repeated requests in the documents he'd sent me, but hadn't seen any answers.

"I sent three requests and all I got were records from two days after the accident. We called the company after the preliminary requests, but by then they said they didn't have copies from back that far." He waved his hand and shook his head. "It doesn't matter. The jury is going to feel sorry for Mrs. Bloom. I think we'll do much better focusing on the property owners. I don't need to remind you that there were over a dozen other cars that had crashed through the storefront over the years, one just four months before yours and the same bakery was smashed into eight years ago. The owners were asked to put up barriers. They had sufficient warning.

"I've met with three witnesses from the scene," he continued, "and located an expert witness who'll testify to the inherently dangerous parking situation at the shopping center. Hopefully that won't backfire. He's an academic type without much work in the real world."

It bothered me that our simple request for the cell phone records of the driver could not be found for that day. It opened up an alternative reason for the accident quite different from a seizure: not paying attention to what one is doing and putting a car into forward rather than reverse. This thought would not go away, though I said nothing more about it that day. "I still don't understand why they were allowed to see all of my therapists' records. We're only suing for physical damages."

"Like I told you, it's the law. If you're suing someone for any damages they can look at all your records."

"Ready to go? We'll be taking Mrs. Bloom's deposition first, and then yours. The Forrests will be last."

The depositions were held in a large conference room overlooking a different part of the city. I had never given a deposition before and was curious about the process. Even more so, I was curious to discover what it would feel like to finally meet the faces and bodies behind the names of the people that I was suing. Ted, Mary, and I were the first to arrive. The Blooms came in shortly afterwards. Mrs. Bloom was a petite woman about my age, who looked like she weighed all of a hundred pounds. She wore a tailored, dark, straight skirt that came just above her knees, and a long sleeved ivory colored blouse that had a shimmer to it. Pale stockings covered her thin legs, and her feet were covered by tidy, little, flat shoes. Dark brown, neatly cut straight hair came down to her shoulders and framed her pinched face with a furrowed, frightened brow. Her eyes were red and swollen from tears, her posture hunched, and lips quivering. She was tearful throughout the proceedings and comforted by her husband, a small but well-built man.

Curious testimony came up. Mrs. Bloom said she didn't know that I was injured until an article appeared in the local paper months later, describing the lawsuit that I had filed. Then she burst into tears describing how it felt to have her name in the paper like that and have herself portrayed like some drunk or something.

I found it hard to believe that she was unaware she'd injured me. I'd spoken with a mutual acquaintance shortly after the accident and had also received flowers from the Blooms while I was in the hospital. Mrs. Bloom seemed more concerned about how she was perceived by the community than she was about my injury, and it took conscious effort to feel some compassion for her.

I looked for something in common. I, too, had felt my

Chapter 16: First Response

self-image violated by the article about my lawsuit, complete with the amount that we were seeking. I didn't want to be viewed as a greedy woman suing someone. We all have our images that we want to protect. I knew that feeling.

Mrs. Forrest presented the perfect contrast. Tall, erect posture, sturdy build, perhaps a generation older than me, calm and smiling something of a Buddha smile. She wore leggings and a tunic. Her shoes were flat, tie shoes, similar to my own. Like Mrs. Bloom, she was accompanied by her husband. He was a taller, rounder man who wore shorts, despite it being January. The Forrests were about the age of my parents, and though they did not resemble them particularly, there were enough similarities that I could not look at them without some feelings of kindness and respect.

I don't remember what I was wearing that day, probably a pair of jeans with a long-sleeved knit shirt and a fuzzy vest. In contrast to Mr. Forrest, I am always cold and wear as many under-layers and over-layers as possible. Frank did not accompany me. He may have been at work, or he may have been at home. He hadn't volunteered and I hadn't felt that I needed him there while I answered a bunch of questions.

Before my own testimony was taken, Ted called the defendant's lawyers into a separate room to discuss a few issues. This was an information-gathering deposition, and as such, anything went; the lawyers were free to ask what color underwear you had on if they thought it might be remotely relevant to their case. Ted was quite concerned that my abortion would come up and could work against us. "All we need is one right-to-lifer on the jury and our case is shot." His fears being what they were, we had agreed to pursue my case solely on the basis of my physical injuries. However, that in itself would not stop the other lawyers from questioning me about other issues without prior agreement.

Ghostwoman

Ted discussed with the attorneys the fact that due to the emotional issues of the case, my license had been suspended and I had not been allowed to work since the previous April. He would agree to not try the case for economic damages related to my emotional issues if they would agree not to bring any of them to light.

Subsequently, my questioning by both of the defendants' attorneys was quite civil, friendly, lacking any twinge of animosity, and no reference was made to any of my history unrelated to my physical injuries.

12-7

Frank came home from work in a happy frame of mind. Greeted by Mondeau, she always brings out his playful side. He told us of a patient he'd seen today who had missed or had been late for 32 appointments! Iyra asked if it was her. We laughed. We're only up to 4.

Though the patient was one hour late, with no one afterwards, he removed her mouthful of rotting teeth. The family discussion shifted into negative judgment about this not-particularly-together patient. I encouraged compassionate thinking about the woman and her life.

Tonight I find myself steering our family conversation into awareness of gratitude and opportunities for giving. I feel self-conscious talking about these things; like I am naked and everyone is staring at me. Now that's something to let go of!

I look at Frank with love and longing, remembering last night when I crawled into bed. He was so warm and smelled so good. His hands caressed mine. Even asleep he was loving me. He cleans the

Chapter 16: First Response

kitchen and talks playfully with the kids. I like this background music, leaving them all in good hands, each others, as I return to my computer and my work.

Later, Frank put the kids to bed while I wrote. Tired, I followed not much later. I am cold, as usual. My hands and feet like ice.

You are like a furnace. Our temperature differential has always helped to keep us together. No matter how upset I am with you, you are so warm and inviting in bed.

I burrow into your side for warmth. I intertwine my icy legs with your warm fuzzy ones. My hands are warmed by the fire of your belly. You are not asleep. You enjoy my cooling influence and take the opportunity to burrow into me with love. We can not seem to kiss each other deeply enough this night.

12-10

Yesterday was nice. A pastel morning sky, an easy temperature, but no time for "Australia," our family code word for my office when I'm writing. "If anyone calls and wants to talk to me, just tell them I'm in Australia."

Doesn't look like there will be much time for writing today either. I've got to get the packages sent off to the family if they can hope to receive them by Christmas, let alone Hanukkah. Then there's the acupuncture appointment and a brief visit to my old job for their holiday potluck. They don't know that I'm leaving, and I wanted a chance to say good-bye and to tell them in my own words where I

Ghostwoman

have been and why I'm not coming back. I'll miss them.

... able to only finish one package, which made it hastily into my car, before calling Thomas to flush out our latest response to the Board. I did not want to be as subtle as he. I wanted them to see their discrimination clearly and acknowledge it.

...A short spin of writing, interrupted by depositions for the bakery crash trial...

...Returning from the depositions, I needed a nap before beginning my holiday letter. I typed for three straight hours, watching the pageant of the year flowing effortlessly. I think I'm too wordy these days. Writing can do that.

There's so much to get done before we leave for California, Christmas at Grandma's. She and Oma are so delighted we can spend the holiday with them. All of Franks brothers and sisters will be down with their families. We haven't all been together since Susan's funeral. I hope it goes well.

Frank stepped in to say hi when he came home from work, and the strangest thing happened. I saw his aura. I hadn't been practicing the type of non-looking that had allowed me to perceive people's energy fields for a while, so it startled me. And it was in the shape of a halo, a halo of pure white light. I'd never seen anything like that before.

Chapter 17
Rage

As always, Eve met us at the airport with a radiant smile, though there was a palpable tension in the air. Frank had blown up at her the last time we'd visited, and my relationship with Eve was still fragile and unpredictable. I had visited her briefly with the kids during the summer, and it had been a beautiful and nurturing three days. But the capacity for our relationship to shift completely was unnerving. I could only share her delight with having us all together, with great unspoken anxiety.

We were the first of the out-of-towners to arrive, and in the warmth of the late afternoon, the kids wheeled their bags into Grandma's house, where they would soon be joined by Frank's sister and her family. After settling them in, Frank and I wheeled our suitcases around the corner to let Oma know we'd arrived. We chose to sleep where the undercurrents in the air were not so thick, and where we could bring Oma a piece of happiness just by being there.

The day after we arrived, Eve treated us to a visit to the new aquarium. It was not crowded, and in that serene and beautiful environment, we were all filled with such awe for the creatures, that it kept us peaceful. Frank's sister, Irmi, and her family arrived that evening, and with the laughter of the children and our joy at seeing one another, I became hopeful for a better Christmas than the two previous years.

The following morning, I awoke to find Oma already at work in her kitchen. She had cleaned the countertop and sprinkled it with powdered sugar, and was taking out the cookie dough she had prepared the day before. She moved adeptly, and with excitement, but her brow was pinched with nervousness. "Just don't tell Eve," she said to me in her heavy accent. "She doesn't vont me to be doing this and if she finds out, I'm going to get it!" Her expression would have sounded humorous had there not been a painful truth behind her words. She and Opa had long been the target for Eve's suppressed emotions. They could do little right in Eve's mind, and were the subjects of numerous chastisements and controlling behaviors. After Opa died, Oma carried this burden alone.

How could we not tell Eve when we were going to be bringing the kipful over for everyone to eat? "We could say that I baked them," I said, watching from the side as Oma deftly rolled out the dough and taught me how to fill them and roll them into their cute little crescent shapes all dusted with powdered sugar. Two pans were done before I walked over to say good morning to the full house at Eve's place.

The sounds of playful cousins reached me from the sidewalk as I approached. My seven-year-old nephew let me in, grabbing a cookie as I carried the rest of them into the kitchen, where Eve was making apple pancakes. "Sorry I'm late, we were baking some kipful. Oma is so happy baking the cookies and seems so energized having a purpose."

"She shouldn't be doing that, Harriet, and I don't need you encouraging her!" Eve snapped, drawing her brows together to make her point.

Chapter 17: Rage

"Why are you so angry? I did most of the work and Oma just told me what to do."

"She's going to get sick now from overdoing it! You all think you know what's best for Oma but you're not around when she gets sick! You don't know anything! Who do you think you are coming in like this?!!"

We all had other ideas about what made Oma sick, but we would not be around to help once we'd gone back to our homes. I drew back, knowing from past experiences that it was pointless to argue with Eve when she started in this way, it just escalated her irrational behavior and made it harder on Oma. So I followed Oma's pleas to not respond to Eve and just let it go. I changed the subject and shifted my attention to playing with the kids and talking with Irmi.

12-23

New blood arrived last evening. The Canadians are here! A tense truce was called between Eve and me. She's just sort of ignoring me and that's better than criticizing everything I say and do. Later I found my little book, *The Art of Peace*. I read it, trying to understand the rhythm of war, or attack, and trying to understand the rhythm of peace, yet not submission to anger, and fear, and hurtful behavior. How to allow feelings, yet use them in a controlled way so that they help heal and do as little harm as possible.

Anger is interesting. I don't ever remember feeling it so clearly before my mystical experience. Before then I felt my anger as sadness and grief. Anger is different. There is this feeling that I become when I let my anger flow, and it is not a bad feeling. It moves stagnant, frustrated energy out of me. It sets boundaries and keeps my emotions flowing forward and not getting stuck. It feels honest, though I have been taught that anger is not an O.K. emotion to reveal. Even mindbody medicine supports restraint in expressing anger towards others, as do all the major religions. How much restraint does creating a world of love require? How much expression of truth?

I suppose the answer is balance and control. To allow oneself to feel the fullness of one's truth, but then to have the capacity to release that truth incrementally and productively, rather than all at once. Like the difference between a bonfire and a bomb.

Though Oma lived for our visits, she eventually stopped coming around to Eve's place to be with all her great-grandchildren. She'd gotten her fill of scowling looks, reprimands, and commands regarding what she was and wasn't allowed to do.

Yet the same Eve who could be so emotionally tormenting would go to the added effort of preparing special food for Oma if she knew Oma didn't like what she fixed for the rest of the family. The love that was Eve's essence could not stop bubbling up through the cracks of her broken psyche.

Frank had to get back to work and flew home early. He'd arranged his vacation so that he'd visit for the shortest time possible to see everyone. He knew his mother did best for short visits, and he couldn't tolerate the way she treated Oma.

But the kids and I remembered the good times, the vast majority of the time we'd known Eve. We hadn't grown up with the years of experience that shaped Frank's desire to come and go so quickly. We wanted to spend as much time as we could with Grandma, and

Chapter 17: Rage

Oma, and all the aunts and uncles and cousins, so our plane tickets would not return us home for another week.

With Frank gone and Oma rarely coming by, I became the target for Eve's pain. I tried in vain to gently talk to her about it, then I let the jabs float by. For days I attempted to ignore the barrage of contradictions and invalidations as I reflected on compassion, remembering the trauma Eve had endured as a child, and reminding myself of the boundless love she had showered on us for years before Susan's death. I tried to imagine how the death of a daughter must feel. I focused my attention on all the care and nurturing Eve still gave to us despite her brokenness.

Until one morning I erupted.

"Enough!" I screamed, and once my voice was found, it did not stop. My voice moved through my body like a tornado, propelling me into the kitchen where I grabbed Eve's shoulders and yelled directly to her face, "Stop trying to hurt me! Stop with the criticisms and the insults! Stop trying to pick fights with me!"

"I'm sorry I've lost my patience!" I continued with a voice that was louder than I ever imagined it could be. "I'm sorry you've been hurt so badly in the past that you can't stop hurting others!"

Then, with my truth revealed in the only way it was able, I walked out of the kitchen into the adjoining living room, shaking.

I took a deep breath, observing what had come over me. "I'm sorry," I calmly stated, wondering how a person could become something so alien to what she knows herself to be.

"No you're not," she rebuked from the kitchen.

"Yes I am. I'm sorry that any of this needed to happen."

A sister-in-law came to console me. "I've been wanting to do that for years," she whispered. The other one could hardly look at me, and let me know she did not think I set a very good example for the children.

"You're probably right," I agreed. "But at least they'll know it's not OK to allow others to abuse you without doing something about it."

Surrendering to love does not mean surrendering to the tyranny of others.

> Fight fire with water, say my books on peace. Fine. But what if there isn't enough water, or the fire is raging out of control? Isn't it controlled firebreaks that are most helpful in these circumstances? Though I'd hardly classify my outburst as controlled. I've never exploded like that before! And to do so on Eve, who I care about so deeply— Where did it come from? Was it my cumulative pent up frustrations, not just with Eve, but with the Board? With Frank? With all the above? These things hardly seem significant enough to account for my degree of rage. I wonder whether there are deeper and more terrible things in my psyche that I can't remember, things in the transpersonal realm, or past life issues smoldering beneath the surface. What I know of myself is so little. Like the tip of an iceberg, most of who we are lies hidden.
>
> Wherever it came from, I am humbled by my inability to control my rage and communicate it a little more delicately.
>
> ... The Paradox arises; never gone, circumstances merely giving it a rest. How to be true to the self. How to honor the self, and honor the other and the whole at the same time? Or maybe I just did?

Chapter 17: Rage

I learned something important this trip. I learned that when we don't speak up for the little hurts, when we don't honor our feelings and take care of ourselves, it builds. And it either explodes, or it can eat away at us slowly.

Mindbody cancer theory notices this— how long-held resentment is associated with higher incidences of cancers. I remember the comments from various attending physicians about cancer patients: how it always hits the nicest people. And what about all those saints who died of throat cancer? Seems like blocked energy in the expression of truth chakra to me. Hmmmm.

We do no one any favors by letting them take advantage of us. When to intervene? If we are honest with ourselves, and listen to our hearts, we know. Just a little kinder next time, please.

In Kabbalah, the fifth level of the Sefirot, the Tree of Life— Justice balanced with Compassion. Not just balancing, but justice emerging FROM compassion; compassion for oneself. AND others.

Thank you Eve. Thank you for reminding me who I am, and what I still need to understand and stand up for. Thank you for showing me hidden places in my heart. And thank you for reminding me why we try to avoid war in the first place. It takes too many generations after a war is over for it to stop.

After three more days of "vacation" we returned home, where I found another version of the Corrective Action Order waiting for me. The Board asked us to respond by the following Tuesday, but as it was New Year's Eve weekend, I wouldn't be able to get in touch with Thomas until that Monday morning. The Board's quarterly meeting was on January fifteenth, and my case was scheduled for discussion at that time. If I found the new order to be acceptable, and signed and returned it by that date, the investigation would be resolved. If not, the Board would consider further action.

The new version of the Corrective Action Order had significant improvements, notably the dropping of the requirement to show the order to prospective employers and to require my supervisor to send quarterly reports to the Board. However, the Board still refused to portray a balanced picture of the varied opinions of my experience, preferring only to document the opinions that I either suffered from bipolar disease or an unspecified mood disorder. They also did not remove the clause, "**...Licensee neither admits or denies a violation of the medical practice act...**"
And they gave themselves sole discretionary power to require me to continue psychiatric monitoring after one year, at my continued expense, of course.

Once again, I could not sign the order.

Thomas sent our response, thanking the IC for the few changes they'd made. Then he delineated the rest of the issues we'd highlighted the first time. He signed it,
   "Very truly yours, Thomas E. McDermott"

Why is it that lawyers can write to each other, even when on opposing sides, and sign off "very truly yours" but a physician who has empathy and compassion for her patients can't sign a chart note "love" without making everybody nervous?

I went to my old clinic to clean out my office that day. It was chilly so I wore a hat Eve crocheted for me years ago. My heart pounded nervously as I descended into the fog and drove slowly along the familiar path. I'd

Chapter 17: Rage

dreamt about leaving my job the night before. It was an uneasy dream. I was feeling incompetent, and deservedly so. I glanced through a chart and noticed a glaring mistake I had made. No wonder they wanted me gone. I packed my things, finding only stuffed animals to take home. I had no books.

Such was not the case in my office, where coworkers stopped by to say hello and goodbye, and share their sorrow that I was leaving. In my real world, there were plenty of books and papers, no stuffed animals, a few artistic tokens from my patients: the planter box that Virginia built and painted for me with the jade and spider plants, and what about the embroidered wall hanging her daughter had made? I'd just gotten it framed and it looked so nice up on the wall. Ruby's painted glass stood on my second floor window bearing flowers that never needed watering.

What to do with all the stuff that held so much love and affection?

Folders were emptied into the recycling bin along with notebooks not consulted in years, unlikely to be looked at again. But what if someone wanted to compare the state of ever-changing "knowledge" over a span of twelve years? I kept 1994 and beyond, along with my old files of diseases. Old mail that had not been forwarded to me, but stuffed into a drawer months ago, awaiting my imminent return, was added to a box. My bulletin board was emptied: taking down my license, my children's' photos, sweet cards, and a napkin with quotes about kindness and love that I collected during the last few days of my work. Carefully I packed them all away, feeling the tenderness I had for my old clinic, my work, my colleagues, and my patients. I would miss them all.

I tried to take my name plate from the door but it wouldn't budge. Ah well. That and my picture in the entryway would remain until the clinic removed them.

The phone rang late that afternoon. It was Dr.

Greenbaum returning my call from earlier in the day. I'd gotten his name from one of the physicians at the Holistic Medical Association conference. "Thanks for getting back to me so quickly. I have an unusual situation and need to find a Board-approved psychiatrist to monitor my mental status." I went on to explain briefly about the meditative experience and how it had gotten the Board so involved in my life. I reviewed the various psychiatrists I had worked with, then explained what it looked like the Board was going to require of me.

"So why aren't you going to be monitored by Dr. Paltrow?" he asked.

"The investigative committee didn't like his assessment and let me know that he wouldn't be acceptable."

I'd specifically asked about Dr. Paltrow at the hearing. One of the members of the committee responded that he would not work out as my monitoring psychiatrist. "Why?" I asked. He answered that we'd discuss it later, but it slipped my mind, so they never had to openly state the reason behind their prejudice.

"My question for you is whether or not you believe that one can have a spiritual experience with an altered state of consciousness that is not necessarily evidence of mental pathology?"

"Well, that would depend, and I'd probably have to see you for at least four visits to make a diagnosis."

Four visits! I hung up shortly afterwards, not wanting to waste any more of his time. I'd need to start all over again. What a waste, what a bother! I guessed the Board and I would eventually agree on Dr. Thompson. She at least knew my story, so the updates could be short and sweet.

I imagined my encounter. I would be angry. I *was* angry. Having to see a psychiatrist not of my choosing, whose diagnosis I disagree with, whose impressions I don't trust. What's the point? How could I see her without being angry?

Chapter 17: Rage

I cried softly before running out to pick up Iyra from swim team.

January 13

Antsy and short-tempered, I've needed to put aside my writing and deal with household affairs. Writing releases so much of my tension and brings me such joy. I had meetings the last two evenings, and another two tonight and tomorrow. I'm the absentee mother, and Frank is doing just fine as the present father. The kids seem to relate better to him than they do to me these days. He still knows how to play, while I busy myself with community work in my attempt to help make the world a better place.

I've always liked community work. The meetings are OK and the people are wonderful. I'm just feeling greedy about not having enough time to work on my own creations.

Came home from the school meeting last night and Frank was reading a book to the kids upstairs. Jade was sitting on Frank's back giving him a massage in exchange for being read to. I had looked in Jade's homework folder before heading up the stairs and noticed he hadn't done any of his homework.

"Oh, no! I forgot!" he exclaimed in raw honesty.

"He told me he didn't have any homework," Frank added.

"Lights out now. You need to get up early to do it in the morning."

Ghostwoman

Jade set his alarm for 6 am, taking the responsibility for getting himself up. How surprised I was to awaken at 6:15 and discover that all his homework was done! Said he woke up around 4:45 and finished all of it immediately. By 6:15 he was ready to watch cartoons.

January 18, Monday
Martin Luther King Day. No school. The kids honored this peaceful man by fighting about the Nintendo game that they were playing. I reminded them of the limit I had imposed on electronic games the day before, thirty minutes followed by two hours of analog life. Then I gave them a project to do before I left for my yoga class. With the help of our puppets, they were to create skits about conflict, and how to resolve it nonviolently...

Jan. 19
'Honor the good things you want for yourself, since desire is the path to God' Deepak Chopra. I think how this quote can be misperceived, but I like it anyway. Fulfilling our desires in an environmentally sustainable manner can help to fulfill another as well. Our desire can create work for others, ideally work that is enjoyed. Creating avenues for money to flow keeps the economy alive. Keeps people feeling worthwhile if they are doing work they believe in.

Very different from satisfying one's desires at the expense of another's happiness. One person's success need not mean another's failure. If we stop

Chapter 17: Rage

being greedy, there is room for all of us to succeed abundantly.

My writing was interrupted by a call from Thomas with the latest update from the Board. They had rejected our most reasonable request for this all to be over if I was psychiatrically cleared after one year. The Board demanded that it remain at their discretion whether or not I was through with them.

Thomas was furious.

"Thomas, there's a little issue of time which I discovered in the small print. If a physician goes more than one year without practicing medicine, they're required to take a one-day computerized exam before being allowed to practice again. I've been practicing a very limited scope of medicine for the last twelve years, which might make my passing such an exam rather difficult. I know my limits and don't take care of hospitalized or emergency cases, but for all I know, the test covers all that and more. My boss has agreed to keep me on as an on-call provider. I want to wrap this up and get back to some work before a year has passed.

"I can agree to the Board's requirement that they have the authority to continue to follow up on me after one year, as long as the other changes that we requested in the document are made. I just can't sign a document that portrays only the opinions of those who think that I suffer from a serious mental illness. And I can't sign a document that insinuates that I may have violated the medical practice act. That's hogwash. Other than that, I can live with their need to scrutinize me."

Frank stood at the sink and whipped through the dishes as fast as the rest of us could clear the dirty ones and put the clean ones away.

"Mom, Jade isn't helping!"

"Yes I am! Why'd you just take that plate away from

me that I was about to take to Daddy?"

"Well, hardly! I've put away all the clean dishes and cleared most of the dirty ones while you just dance around!"

" Plllt!" he blew Iyra a raspberry and carried a piece of silverware to the dishwasher.

"I bet you two were married in a past life and argued all the time and were put on earth as brother and sister to learn how to stop bickering," I said. Jade laughed at the thought.

Frank moved into the dining room where he sat at the table in front of his house drawings. He was planning a kitchen remodel and was always happiest when he could be creative.

Iyra picked up her clarinet and practiced at the kitchen table. Jade sang along: "Lou, Lou, skip to my Lou! Skip to my Lou my darling." *Frere Jacques* came next.

From the office I could hear Iyra stop playing and start yelling, "Stop it, Jade! Stop it!"

I walked quietly in and found him moving and making faces to the music.

"Iyra, it's a compliment that he can't sit still to your playing."

"I don't care! He's bothering me and I need to practice and I want him to go away!"

He stuck his tongue out at her and she chased him around the house with her clarinet.

Thomas called the following day. "Harriet, I spoke with the attorney for the Board today and clarified our issues. He seems fine with including the opinions of all the psychiatrists and agreed to leave out the line about you neither admitting or denying."

"Finally!"

"He should be sending me the papers in the next day or two. I'll have my secretary call you when they arrive so you can sign them."

Chapter 17: Rage

Unfortunately, the papers that Thomas received did not include the changes that were agreed upon over the phone. They still included only the opinions of the psychiatrists who chose to label my experience as a symptom of a major mental illness.

Thomas deftly rewrote the order on official Oregon Board of Medical Examiners' stationary, including the opinions of my mental health allies, as well as the results of the psychological testing. Then he signed it and sent it back to the attorney for the Board to either sign, or to file an appeal.

While Thomas was writing letters on my behalf to the Board, I was sending a letter to Eve, trying, yet one more time, to both let her know she is loved, and help her see how hurtful her behavior was. She returned my effort with a letter of her own. It was a kind letter that lacked the drama and negativity that our Christmas interactions contained, but nothing was resolved. It did not include an apology or any acknowledgment of a problem with her behavior. Still, I was grateful the communication between us continued. As long as there is communication there is a thread of hope, and love can weave its healing ways.

January 22

Another day of cold and dreary rain, eclipses for Shabbat in SNOW! Beautiful Snow!!! The children dance like snowflakes!

Frank, too, seems delighted. Despite his head wound from this morning's leap over the last three steps and headfirst into the ceiling beam, he has been in a most happy mood tonight. He wrestles with the kids and their laughter is the background music for my writing and my household office work.

Ghostwoman

January 28th

I have no patience today. I awoke a little blue, tired, went back to bed after straightening up the house. What a mess. The kids' floors were covered with dirty clothes, garbage, clean clothes, blankets, books, toys, and a few you-name-its. My life feels like an endless rerun of clean up, only to be messed up again. I clean muddy dogs only to have them want to go right back out again. So much mirrors a feeling of endless purposeless movement. Fixing a water main one year, only to have to do it again the next. Fixing an oven, only to have to go through it five more times within a year. Writing pages one day, only to find them pointless and heading in the wrong direction the next day; I delete them all. Finding supportive professional literature that validates my experience, only to have it ignored.

What is it that makes an action feel fulfilling one day, yet futile the next? Lack of (enough) patience and validation, perhaps. Expectations for results. Lack of acceptance for Divine will, i.e., acceptance of the perfection (even if in some inconceivable way) of whatever happens. Forgetting that all is in the hands of God, all manifestation IS the hands of God. And those hands are connected to a loving heart.

Clarity takes time. Muddy ponds need to settle. I am grateful for the reassurances of my thumbs. I practice watching my breath, feeling my frustrated emotions; then I let them go.

Chapter 17: Rage

Thomas called with good news, for a change. The Board accepted his rewritten order with the language we insisted upon. Yippee! I took only a few minutes to celebrate my relief, then began wading through the fifteen-page reactivation packet I'd set aside on my desk. My tango with the Board was coming to a close.

Similarly, my accident case was approaching its court date resolution.

Frank and I, however, were nowhere near resolving our problems. Still becoming more fully aware of them, defining who we were and working with our relationship became the central drama of our life.

I interpreted the way the mystical experience followed my decision to leave Frank, completely altering that desire, to mean that the highest will of God was for Frank and me to stay together.

Yet in the day-to-day world of our relationship, part of me died every time my heart went unheard, every time I asked for something so small that meant so much to me and seemed impossible for him.

Through pain, I became clearer and clearer about my essential need for words and actions that expressed caring, as well as my need to discover and express my truth as kindly as possible, even when that truth included anger. As one who cared for others, I too needed to be filled with love, to be replenished. Hugs and affection, expressed appreciation and concern, soul time, quiet time, intellectually stimulating time, different things at different times, but as long as we give, we will need. In the endless cycle of inhaling and exhaling, it is up to each of us to learn what we need to breathe in that is sustaining, allowing us to give back again and again.

In the mystical experience, the direct connection to the Source of all love filled me completely. However, in my day-to-day existence of ordinary consciousness, I was part of a web of relationships, manifestations of the One, that helped fill each other's needs. I call this functional codependency, the interconnectedness of people and of all things, breathing for and with each other. Like plants and animals, breathing out what each other needs to breathe in.

Within this great web, each relationship needs to stand in its own integrity. The strength of the whole rests on the structure of each strand. Cleaning up one individual relationship or situation cannot clean up another. So with the Board situation moving behind me, it was time for Frank and me to resume working on our mess.

Chapter 18
Unconditional Love

Lauri had told me about a lecture titled, *Your Body is Talking, Are You Listening?* I had mentioned the talk to Frank, who thought it sounded interesting, and I was quite surprised when the opportunity to play poker with his buddies came up that same night, and Frank elected to go late to the game so that he could attend a talk about the emotional connection between illness and health. It felt wonderful to be sharing an interest together. We hadn't talked about mindbody issues since he'd returned from the Tibetan medical conference and I hoped this would be a place where our relationship could find something meaningful in common.

It was dusk as I drove us to the presentation, and for most of the way we had little to say to each other. I was building my courage to ask Frank if he wouldn't mind taking out my stitches from the surgery I'd had ten days before. My leg had been bothering me, so I had the two upper screws removed when Frank was at work and the kids were at school. None of them had inquired about how the procedure had gone and I hadn't brought it up.

Ginger, who was still living in our basement, had driven me to the hospital.

Lauri picked me up and took me home, first taking me to her house for some homemade soup, and an ice pack; insisting on giving me the nurturing that I so needed and could hardly ask for.

"Its simple," Frank responded to the request I finally got out. "You should do it yourself. It's just your leg and you can reach it easily enough."

"Fine," I snapped, feeling hurt, "then I'll do it myself."

"You don't have to get mad. People get better when they take responsibility for their own healing."

"It just would have felt nice," I said, not knowing what else to say, afraid to remind him that people heal the best when they feel appreciated and cared about.

We said nothing to each other after that, for a bit. Frank's remark sent me wanting my distance from him and wishing I hadn't invited him along. He was the first to speak, asking me what kind of anesthesia I had. He was trained in anesthesiology and had used both I.V. and oral anesthesia on his dental patients over the years.

"I had I.V. sedation," I answered, feeling the storm about to burst. "I mentioned your recommendation for oral sedation and local anesthesia to my orthopedist, but he said it had been his experience that the screw removal went more smoothly and comfortably with I.V. medication."

"What a waste of money! The whole anesthesia thing is political. You didn't need the I.V. sedation and it costs ten times as much. You have to pay the anesthesiologist and for all that equipment. It was a big waste of time and money for your procedure and oral medication would have been quite sufficient."

"The insurance paid for most of it."

"That's not the point. The higher the cost of care, the more it drives up insurance costs. I told you, you didn't

Chapter 18: Unconditional Love

need the I.V. sedation."

"Would you please get off my case about it!? The surgery went fine."

We spoke no more for the rest of the short drive. Frank was angry about my not following his suggestions, and I was fuming about his greater concern for politics and perhaps his pride, than for my well-being. By the time we arrived at the lecture and found the room where our talk was going on, I sat down and Frank sat down one seat away from me.

The flyers on the chairs said, **"Love. Love is not measured by how many times you touch each other but by how many times you reach each other."**

With great effort, I moved next to Frank.

Dr. Martin, a middle aged man with a hefty belly, was already talking by the time we had found the room. He had just begun and was giving a brief history of his life, with pertinent facts that brought him to his realizations about healing and illness. Years of practice as a therapist and healer had demonstrated to him that illness and healing are a function of the mind. The mind consisted of conscious and unconscious elements, and by knowing the mind and connecting through love, healing could occur. From everything. Even genetic illnesses and defects, degeneration of the body, depression, premature aging; you name it, he'd seen it. And between my personal experience of the world being simultaneously a sea of consciousness and love, and writings about the healing abilities of highly consciously evolved humans, it made sense to me that anything was possible.

Dr. Martin talked about the spiritual plane, its relationship to our minds, and its consequent effect on our health. He talked of past lives and karma to our group as if it were as generally accepted as good nutrition and exercise.

The stories of his experiences validated all the knowledge that was shared with me during my mystical experience. He even gave the example of allergies being the result of belief and programming from the level of the mind, and hence, treatable from the perspective of psychospirituality.

I remembered my patient with allergies and her negative reaction to my sharing similar thoughts. We have to be so careful about how, and to whom, we present this sort of information.

Like me, Frank was very interested in the talk and suggested we sign up for private healing sessions over the weekend. We walked out talking to each other again, both of us excited about the information we had just heard; and me, excited that Frank was just as interested in this as I was, hoping that Dr. Martin could work some miracles on us as well.

The following day was a cold, rainy morning, but the threat of ice had temporarily moved on. I was looking out the back window at the dogs when Frank came back from driving to pick up Iyra's friend. He was about to go down into the garage to remove the studded tires and put the regular tires back on my car. Mondeau and Ginger's dog, Akela, who had been living with us since Ginger had moved into our basement, were wrestling on the little slope above the deck. Between the plumbing and the dogs, what had been a soft grassy area surrounded by perennial beds was now a swath of solid gray-brown mud. Akela kept stepping in the perennials, then the dogs frolicked over to the vincas below the bay tree and continued to wrestle near our muddy springs.

"How do you do it?" I asked Frank. "How do you keep your cool with two dogs that dig up the yard and trammel the garden that you've just spent months tending? And the dogs get filthy! They're coated with mud! Even their eyeballs are muddy from sticking their

Chapter 18: Unconditional Love

heads into the mud holes they've created."

Frank just smiled warmly. "This is as good as it gets," he said calmly as we watched the dogs together.

"What do you mean, this is as good as it gets? Ongoing drudgery of cleaning muddy dogs that have torn up the garden, only to let them back out to do it all over again?"

Frank and the kids were smitten with Mondeau, but dogs were never my thing. Mondeau was the best, and was teaching me to love dogs, but they always seemed to want attention when I wanted to put my attention elsewhere. They need to go out. They need to come in. Leaving them in their fairly large outdoor pen was not an option for me since it made Mondeau so sad.

"It's as good as it gets," Frank repeated. "This is a lesson in something. If it wasn't the dogs and the garden, it would be something else, and perhaps something not nearly as wonderful as the dogs and the garden. You just do your best at enjoying the gardening and cleaning the dogs."

We watched the two dogs together for a while. They were on the side of the yard by the tall deciduous trees, next to the fence. Mondeau was furiously digging her hole while Akela lay in the mud, watching. Akela looked over at Frank and me. I wondered what her look meant. Was she remembering my screaming at her thirty minutes ago to get out of the raised vegetable beds on the other side of the house? Or just before then, when I yelled at her to get out of the hardy (before we had two dogs living with us) geraniums? Was she afraid to dig anywhere? Was that necessarily bad? I thought of my own fears to do what I thought was fun, and felt sorry for ruining her joyful pastime. She turned her attention over to Mondeau's hole, then stood up and joined in the digging fray. Before long, she was digging in the deep hole while Mondeau's head and forelegs poked between Akela's legs, then from that ridiculous position, Mondeau started digging a different hole of her own. Akela's digging showered Mondeau's wet and muddy head with yet another mountain of dirt and mud.

Frank and I began howling with laughter. "It's an O.K. place to be digging," Frank reassured me. "They're dogs. They dig. The moles are getting active and they're going after them."

Later, after the rains had washed one of the layers of dirt off, Frank cleaned the dogs enough before carrying them, one at a time, up the stairs and into the bath. I offered to help, but he was quite happy to do the job with the girls while I continued my writing before starting dinner.

We still had a mud hole for a garden. We still had two golden retrievers to tend to in Oregon rain, but somehow it was better. We had laughed together.

I had great hopes for our appointments with Dr. Martin, the following day, but neither Frank nor I had a particularly eventful session with him. What I did get from the session was the opportunity to meet Kate, the owner of the house where Dr. Martin was doing his sessions. She held weekly meditations at her home, and invited me to join their meditation circle.

About a week later I decided to take Kate up on her invitation, but I'd misplaced her phone number. Remembering that they met on Tuesdays, I decided to just drop by. She lived less than a mile away, so if this night didn't work out, I could at least get her number again for another time.

When Frank came home from work, I put the lasagna I'd fixed on the table, then told him and the kids where I was headed for the evening. I didn't want to be late and asked them to save some dinner for when I came home.

"How long do you think you'll be?" Frank asked.

"I don't know, a couple hours I imagine." Then I kissed them all good-bye and headed for the door, feeling

Chapter 18: Unconditional Love

that light, delicious blend of nervousness and excitement that only spontaneity can bring.

It was a chilly night, with snow falling lightly. I drove carefully up to Kate's home in the winding hills, and quietly knocked on the door. It turned out that they were meeting at another home for meditation that night, and I was invited to join them. They were also going to be studying the Mayan calendar, something I'd heard about at the Wholeness Center, but had never looked into, so it sounded very interesting.

The house was a half hour away, and between study, meditation, and visiting, the evening took far longer than I anticipated. I considered calling at one point, but thought Frank might be asleep and I did not want to wake him. He had once told me that he didn't worry about me— he didn't worry about much of anything for that matter— so I didn't think the call was necessary. I was more concerned with making him angry by waking him up. It was eleven-thirty when I returned home.

"Where were you?" asked Frank, still awake, eyes glaring. "You said you were just going to be gone for a couple hours! You told us to save you some dinner for when you came home!"

"It lasted longer than I thought it would. Why are you still up?"

"Waiting for you. Why didn't you call?" he answered, still glaring.

"By the time I realized it was getting late, I was afraid I'd wake you. Besides, you've told me before that you don't worry about me."

"I don't," he snapped. "But Iyra did. She wouldn't let me go to sleep. You didn't leave a number. I even drove over to the house looking for you but no one was there."

"I'm really sorry," I said sincerely. "Tonight they went over to some friends' house on the east side for their meditation circle and they invited me to join them."

Frank said nothing more. He shot me one last bitter

Ghostwoman

glance then turned around and went upstairs to bed.

Next time I'll call, I thought to myself, no matter what time it is. Then I lingered downstairs with a cup of tea and my new Natural Time Calendar, happy to be with something that inspired positive thoughts and feelings, rather than Frank's anger.

The calendar, a modern application of ancient Mayan wisdom, followed the rhythms of both the sun and the moon, like the Jewish calendar. I was intrigued, wondering how much of the symbols and meanings I was looking at were truly part of the Mayan civilization, how much was channeled information, and how much was a creation of New Age imagination. The symbol meanings all supported an expansive feeling of benevolence and creativity. Strength, truth, vision, synchronicity, freewill, and more. I tried to backtrack the process that one of the fellows had followed to identify my personal galactic signature. He uncovered it from the combined energies of my birthday. I am a tone #3, Yellow Electric Warrior, whatever that means.

The following evening we all sat down to dinner together. I'd had a good day! Fixed my printer problem, took a yoga class in the morning, then finished up the tobacco talks I'd volunteered to give to the sixth grade science classes. I even found a spot of time to look at my new Mayan calendar again, and wondered if the kids would think it was as cool as I did.

I led a blessing with the kids, but before I could ask about anyone's day or tell them about my unusual night, Frank started getting on my case for not keeping a ledger for my business expenses.

"Frank, I hardly have a business. I'm not making any money, I'm just sort of educating myself."

"But you hope to earn money from this stuff. Now's the time to start keeping track of it. Every successful business keeps good records."

"Thank you for sharing that information. I'll keep

Chapter 18: Unconditional Love

track of what I spend on my books and conferences." But I wasn't feeling thankful, a feeling of nervous dread and anger was coming over me.

"And another thing. We only have one income and you seem to be spending money right and left."

"I don't think so! I pay for the kids' camps and their clothes; they grow out of them constantly, you know. For me, all I've spent is for books and a couple of local conferences. Oh, and I eat lunch at cheap restaurants with my friends a few times a month. I've budgeted thirty dollars for that." The tone of Frank's voice was so bitter I began to loose my appetite.

"I can't believe you didn't call last night! That was so thoughtless, Harriet!"

Iyra chimed in, "I was so worried about you. I thought you got into an accident or something since the roads were icy. I was so scared!"

"Look! I said I was sorry about that! How many times do I have to say I'm sorry for the same thing? Iyra, I told Daddy last night and I'll tell you, I promise I'll call next time no matter how late it is. I didn't want to wake you up." And that was that with Iyra. But Frank went on and on.

"Frank, the way you're talking to me hurts," I said firmly. "All you ever seem to do is criticize things I do and harp on my mistakes. I need some balance. I need some positive feedback about something. Anything! All you seem to notice and comment on is what I do wrong or how I'm mistaken about one thing or another. You never thank me or give me emotional support or tell me anything that makes me think you care about me!" At some point I realized I was raising my voice and got up and left the table so that I wouldn't yell at him. I was livid and needed space to calm down.

Frank and I ignored each other the rest of the night.

In the morning, Frank was off to work by a quarter to seven and I woke the kids and got them breakfasted and

Ghostwoman

off to school. I spent the morning in our office, settling our expenses and writing them out so that Frank could plainly see that I was not spending money right and left. I gathered the receipts for my books and my tapes as I was able, then pulled together my "business" expenses and started a little file. It wasn't a bad idea; I just resented the patronizing way he'd recommended it.

Ginger had offered to fix dinner for us that evening, and since our oven was broken again, she'd gotten permission to use our old oven at the Wholeness Center. I gave her my recipe for manicotti, and wrote until the kids came home. Then off we went to the store for last minute Valentine cards for their classes.

Valentines' Day is a last-minute thing around our house. The first few years after Frank and I were together, I'd gotten excited about it and given Frank cards; but he didn't remember or do anything, so after a while, I just ignored it too, except with the kids.

The table was set and I was helping Jade with his cards when Frank came home. He looked like he was clenching his teeth, and his eyes were cold and narrowed. He brushed past me without a hello, heading up to change out of his work clothes. Minutes later he came back downstairs and Ginger bounced in with our hot, oven baked meal.

"Are you going to join us?" I asked her.

"Not tonight. I've got some things I need to catch up on so I'm just going to go down to my little apartment for the night."

"Thanks so much for cooking dinner!"

"It was my pleasure! I even baked a second tray for the Wholeness Center. I'll see you later!" and she disappeared down the hallway.

Frank sat down and pleasantly began talking with the kids about this and that. He said nothing to me, but periodically shot me stern glances.

"Would you like some manicotti?" I asked.

Chapter 18: Unconditional Love

"No thanks," he answered. "I'm not hungry. My stomach is eating me up." He paused before adding, "I don't think I can live with a wife who's always yelling at me."

"Yelling at you? When was I yelling at you?"

"Last night."

"I didn't yell at you! I may have raised my voice a little but I didn't yell at you."

The yelling began to explode inside me. What about what I had been saying last night? Had I been talking to the walls? Couldn't he ever hear that I had some emotional needs?

I suddenly picked up my plate, turned my back on my family and quickly stepped through the little kitchen to the dark green dining room on the other side. It was the darkest room in the house. I could count the times I'd *ever* yelled at Frank on one hand. I rarely raised my voice. I made a point of saying encouraging things, and expressing my gratitude to him. I took one small bite of my dinner and pushed it away.

Frank called after me to come back and talk about it. *Talk* about it? *Talk*? My whole body was shaking, I wanted to scream. I knew I was losing whatever self-control I had left. To talk about it meant to allow Frank to emotionally clobber me!

I dropped my plate on the table and darted through the living room, down the steps to the front door, and out of the house as fast as I could.

It was dark outside. Cool, misty, and windy. I stormed from the house, down the long driveway towards the street. Our neighbor was putting out his garbage. I pulled myself together enough to wave and say a quick hello as I strode past him in the darkness. I wondered if he could see the tears streaming down my cheeks and hoped they were hidden by the night. It didn't really matter. Nothing mattered.

"I can't take it anymore!" I cried to the Universe. "I

can't take the criticisms and the lack of understanding, appreciation, or affection! I've had enough, thank-You!

"Why do You put me through this? Why have You interrupted every reasonable opportunity I've had to leave this relationship? You know what I need, you created me. So why do You make it so hard? Why does it have to feel so empty?"

I walked as quickly as I was able up our hill, on the edge of the narrow road. I could feel the rod in my leg with every step, kicking me in the shin from the inside. "Take me away," I pleaded. Until the kicking, and the cold, and the wet, and the wind on my face gently began cooling me down, slowly calming my frustrations. Coolness. Step by step. Wetness. Kick by kick. Wind blowing wet hair. Explosion over? Exhaling fetid smoke, inhaling cool clean air, exhaling frustrations. Sadness draining from me through my tears.

The night air wrapped itself around me and whittled away the edges of my pain. It felt good to be outside, to be free. By the time I reached the top of the hill my anger had collapsed in upon itself. I could breathe and I could talk, though I felt hopeless about my relationship with Frank. I turned around and headed back towards home.

> I open my heart
> and you sink your teeth into it.
> How can I protect myself
> but to erect walls to keep the pain
> as far away as possible.
> Walls that I have just worked so hard
> to tear down.

I peacefully walked back in the house and brought my plate back to the kitchen table to talk.

Frank said he couldn't handle anyone yelling at him.

I thought about what Frank had told me about

Chapter 18: Unconditional Love

growing up with a mother who unpredictably and uncontrollably would yell at her children, sharing her own scars with those she loved.

"I promise I will never yell at you again," I said to Frank, with pure sincerity and confidence that I could uphold my simple vow. After all, I raised my voice so rarely.

I finished a few bites, then began cleaning up. Frank started talking about what made *him* so upset. "There were three things," he began, and then went on and on about the other night, how I didn't call and had left implying I'd be back in about an hour or so and came home four and a half hours later.

"How many times do I have to apologize for the same thing? Didn't you already tell me last night about this? Didn't I already tell you I'd call the next time?!?"

"You're raising your voice."

"And what about *my* feelings? I tell you about my feelings and what I need and you never acknowledge them. I ask you to balance your criticisms with a little kindness and gratitude for what I do and who I am, but all I hear are criticisms. And now, the same ones repeated over and over again."

Jade put his hands over his ears and left to go up to his room. Iyra hung around at the edge of the kitchen, watching helplessly.

Eventually, like a tidal wave, hopelessness that I could ever be understood and supported swelled up in an enormous wave. I spun around from the sink. Frank was on the other side of the little L-shaped counter. He was pounding me again with his words. It was like that moment with Eve, when something inside of me took over and moved me through space exploding through my voice. I stormed towards Frank with the counter between us. "The only way for us to resolve this is for me to die!" I screamed.

In a fraction of a second Frank threw the wine he was

Ghostwoman

drinking in my face. I felt the glass connecting to the bridge of my nose. It was not a painful sensation, just a startled one, like being hit with a car. Nerves taking their time to register, body pumped full of chemicals of emotion that quiets the brain from feeling anything in particular. A sensation that did not yet begin to hurt. The body taking a back seat to the pain of the soul.

I turned and ran toward the end of the little room, turning back around at the doorway, after hearing the sound of breaking glass behind me. Frank's wine glass lay shattered next to my feet and I watched as he grabbed the heavier water glass and begin to fling it towards the wall by me. Iyra stood next to me, watching, her eyes wide and filled with terror.

I ran from the kitchen around the corner and up the narrow stairs to my bedroom. I could not stop the waves of violent sobbing.

Frank showed up in the doorway.

"Just leave me alone! Go away and leave me alone! It's never going to work out. Our marriage is never going to work out! I am done with this relationship!"

"Stop it! Stop saying that!"

Frank came towards me and held me down, his hand firmly pressed against my mouth, keeping me from saying anything. "You're programming our marriage for failure! Say you want to work it out. Say we CAN work it out."

All I could do was lie there, staring at him, spitting my own venomous glances into his terror-filled eyes. Iyra was standing in the room to the left of Frank's shoulder. "Just say it Mommy," she pleaded, "Just say it!"

"Mmmflmmpf!"

"Daddy, she can't say anything unless you let go of her."

Finally, Frank let go of my mouth, but continued to hold me down by my shoulders.

"We can work it out, but only if you get some help.

Chapter 18: Unconditional Love

Unless you get some counseling I am done with this marriage!" I said emphatically but without yelling, matching the glare in his eyes.

"Me? You're the one who needs counseling to control *your* anger," he retorted.

"My anger? Just look at the kitchen, Frank. Look at the way you're holding me down. Look at me!"

Frank finally let go of my shoulders but I did not move.

"What's your problem with seeing a counselor anyway?" I asked.

"It's none of their business."

"We're not getting anywhere by ourselves. I won't live like this any more."

It was not the intensity of Frank's reaction that was pushing me to leave, again, but the intensity of the pain I felt that made me scream out my despair in the first place. It was similar to that Christmas with Eve and just before the mystical experience. Only this time, I was not rescued by Grace in the form of expanded, blissful consciousness, but rather the experience of Grace as a clarity of emotional truth that was as solid as my bones.

Love was the heart of the mystical experience, and Love was here, too, the love for myself and Frank. It was Love that allowed me to feel my despair; Love that allowed me to scream it when I couldn't be heard otherwise; Love, that allowed me to see the terror in Frank's eyes as he held me down; Love, that spoke of the need to work in a way that was bigger than the two of us; and it was Love that was willing to be a little more patient, to wait for a long time until Frank and I either healed our brokenness together, or came to the realization that we would both be happier apart.

Unconditional Love wasn't about staying in our relationship as husband and wife. Unconditional Love was about honoring our deepest truths and negotiating the most compassionate pathway to get there for both of us; working from our relationship, healing through our relationship, and perhaps changing our relationship so that we could more deeply feel an honest love for one another once again— perhaps as husband and wife, perhaps not.

And God's will in all of this? Through my Judaism, I would eventually remember that the relationship with God is not one of being a passive recipient of God's will, but being in intimate negotiation and relationship. We are not separate from God, but one with God, and as such our thoughts and feelings matter. We are aspects of God becoming. God, growing. God, evolving. God, living. And we are given our limited consciousness and our individual natures, to love, and to choose, and to live in the way that is most uniquely and lovingly true to ourselves. Ideally while living in harmony with the rest of the world.

Though it would take years, I eventually understood that the point of the mystical experience wasn't to keep me in my marriage with Frank, but to show me how good I had the potential to feel, regardless of my relationship with Frank. And the first step to feeling that goodness was following my own breath, not another's, remembering my own desires, and feelings, and making a place for that in my world.

"I'm so grateful you had an opening today," I said to Dr. Bice.

"Me too. I'm worried about you."

"I'll be O.K. He's never done anything like that before and I know he didn't mean to hurt me."

"They never do."

"No, really, I think I'm safe enough. I not only saw his anger that night, but I believe I saw some self-control. He was wild. Could have done a lot more damage than he did. He's strong. Too bad you can't meet him, but I

Chapter 18: Unconditional Love

understand why you don't see couples if you've already established a relationship with one of the pair. It might feel like we're ganging up."

"That, plus I'd hardly be an independent observer. I've heard too much about Frank and have my own biases. But I can recommend some people to you if you need."

"I have the name of someone but she doesn't have any openings for a couple of weeks. I'm just not sure what to do right now. We've got tickets to all go to Hawaii in five days. I signed up for a yoga retreat months ago and I invited the family to join me. Frank overheard me talking to a friend and said that if I was planning to move out after we returned, he and the kids would go somewhere else for vacation."

"So what do you want to do?"

What did I want to do?

After a year of working with David, knowing what I wanted was only slightly clearer than when we began. It was a question made complex by discovering too many levels of who I was, which were far from integrated. Was I the woman with such pain in her relationship she wanted to leave it at any cost? Or was I the woman who saw a pain larger than her own and wanted to stay and help heal the brokenness? Was I the mind before the mystical experience? During it? Afterwards?

Who was the ghostwoman?

At some level, my relationship with Frank seemed to be a part of my purpose here on earth. I sensed something vital to the Universe about healing our relationship, and through that, helping to heal each other and our little corner of the world.

Frank had been such a gift for much of my life. He was the first man, besides my father, who had ever made me feel loved and wanted. He gave me our children, financially supported the family, and when things between us became difficult, he became the inspiration that returned me to a deeper understanding of myself, of consciousness, and God. Frank was also one of the main inspirations to begin my meditation practice, which continued to be my greatest teacher. But we were at a crossroads where I was beginning to feel that who he loved was no longer who I was.

What did I want? I wanted to heal my ego, reunite with my wholeness, and be one with Oneness again. I wanted to be happier, and I wanted Frank to be happy, with or without each other. But that wasn't all. At a level beyond my own little world, I wanted to study consciousness and its relationship to healing. I wanted to be in the world in a deeply healing way.

Returning home after my session with Dr. Bice, I stopped at the bottom of our driveway to pick up the mail. There was a letter from the Board, which I tore open before getting back into the car. My license had been reactivated! It hadn't taken weeks like the urgent papers had said. I smiled deeply for the first time in days, then climbed back into my car and drove the rest of the way up to the house.

These past six days have not all been horrible. Frank helped Jade build his paddle boat for his science fair project two days ago. I helped time the races. Iyra finished her project completely.

I called for clarification today and to hear who the Board requires me to see. Ms. Wong answered my voice mail to the Board's secretary and told me that the Board wanted me to see Dr. Thompson. I placed a call to her, which she returned after a short while. She doesn't think it's advisable to monitor me. I tried to explain that it was the Board who was requiring us to work together, then vented a

Chapter 18: Unconditional Love

little frustration that I wasn't allowed to choose who I wanted.

Dr. Thompson said she'd call the Board and explain that she was unable to take the position requested of her. I asked her to do me a favor, if she could, of recommending that I be allowed to see Dr. Paltrow. She was not sure that she could do that, but she'd think about it.

One down. Time to give Betsy a call to arrange some substitute work at least one day, at least one hour, before the year is out and I need to retake that test. Maybe it doesn't count now that my license has been reinstated, but I want to be sure. Besides, I grow rustier everyday.

I heard Frank talking to the Iyra this morning after she and Jade had been fighting. He was quietly explaining how anger is an afflictive emotion and that Iyra should learn to control it and to have compassion.

Control, yes. Repress, no. Repression is what makes control become so difficult. Emotions are trying to tell us something. But Frank's right about needing to express our feelings with compassion. He seems to have patience and compassion for everyone but me.

I took my wedding ring off today.

I have heard, echoed repeatedly, that the key to happiness is to choose to be happy. When my heart is heavy, it is heavy, and choosing to be happy seems as possible as choosing to be a man if one

Ghostwoman

is a woman, choosing to be a tree when one is a blade of grass, choosing to be a butterfly when one is still a caterpillar, or sadder yet, a confused earthworm.

To align myself with God I listen to my heart and accept it, love it, try to understand it, and pray for the guidance to know how and when to respond to it. I think I know why my heart chooses to feel sadness so many days, but I always seem to be looking outside myself when I find the answer. What is the answer that comes from inside of me? That I can do something about?

I picked up a half-read book sitting next to me: *Stumbling Toward Enlightenment* by Geri Larkin. It opened to a page that began with a quote by Ranier Maria Rilke, *Letters to a Young Poet*.

"Be happy about your growth, in which of course you can't take anyone with you, and be gentle with those who stay behind; be confident and calm in front of them and don't torment them with your doubts and don't frighten them with your faith or joy, which they wouldn't be able to comprehend. Seek out some simple and true feeling of what you have in common with them, which doesn't necessarily have to alter when you yourself change again and again; when you see them, love life in a form that is not your own....."

Thank-you, Geri. Thank-you, Ranier Rilke.

Chapter 19
Loose Ends

I sat in Ted's office, his sleek wooden desk between us looking as big as half my home office. Ted sat behind the desk, round and jolly, looking out at me and the sweeping view of the city beyond the wall of windows to my back. Mary, his assistant, sat next to me.

I was there to be coached for the upcoming trial for the car accident.

"I'm still not convinced she had a seizure, Ted. Why didn't you ask the neurologist any of my questions about pseudoseizures at the deposition?"

"Look, we've been over all of this. I think the jury will feel sorry for Mrs. Bloom and even if they thought she didn't have a seizure, I don't think we'd get much from her. Plus, we signed off on the *Mary Carter* agreement at the settlement hearing; we can't get more than fifty thousand from them no matter what. Besides, *I* think she had a seizure. One of the witnesses saw her tires still spinning after the car had come to a stop and had to reach in and turn off the engine."

"But didn't the other witness claim to have seen the car completely stopped for some time before crashing through the bakery? She'd have had to put it into the wrong gear, and then had her seizure."

"It doesn't matter. It was an accident either way, and our best bet is to go after the Forrests. After all, they had plenty of warnings that there was a problem, a dozen other similar incidents before yours. We have testimony that they were repeatedly asked for posts in front of the building, but never did anything about it. In fact, we have one picture that clearly shows curb stops in front of all the other buildings except the bakery; not that they would have done much to stop the car." Ted spoke with enthusiasm, his hands moving as he spoke, conducting his words into a symphony.

"Let it go; we've got a lot to cover. First, remember not to say anything about insurance; if anyone mentions that word it's an automatic mistrial."

"That's so ridiculous! It's the insurance company that will be paying the settlement. Why can't you mention the truth?"

"It's the law. Now, when you take the stand, I'm going to ask you the same questions that the jury is asked— your name, your age, your occupation, then I'm going to ask you who you live with. Go ahead and give me your answers."

"What do I say about my work? I resigned."

"Didn't you say you still do on-call work for the county? Just say that you work for the county. That'll go well with the jury, knowing you take care of indigent clients."

"My name is Harriet Cohen, I'm forty-two years old. I'm a physician and I work for Multnomah County. I live with my husband and two kids."

"Don't just say two kids; we want the jury to relate to you, to know that you love your kids and know how this accident has affected your life. Give the names and ages of your children."

He continued. "OK, now, how are you feeling today? And tell me exactly how your leg feels."

Chapter 19: Loose Ends

Clearly Ted was not wanting my usual "fine" for an answer. How did my leg feel? I was always trying *not* to think about it. What brought it pain? What made it hurt? And I knew that the worse I felt, the more compensation the jury might award.

I limped out of Ted's office feeling gray and lifeless. Forcing my responses into predictable little packages felt so contrived and unnatural that even speaking truth felt like a lie. Focusing on my limitations and agonies, the exact opposite of thoughts that brought me joy, seemed to make my leg hurt more. My knee was visibly more swollen those days, though perhaps as much from my lack of time to get to my yoga classes with all these lawyer meetings taking place. I just wanted the whole thing to be done with, and kept turning the outcome over to the wisdom of God.

In the end, we settled after only a half-day of the trial, during our lunch break in Ted's spacious office. All we'd accomplished that morning was choosing the jury, opening presentations by the lawyers, and the judge meeting privately with Ted and me in his chambers in an attempt to get us to settle the case. During lunch, the Forrest's attorney, who had been dramatically quaking during his speech (reminding me of myself doing presentations) gave us a call. He was offering a little more compensation, something he had not budged on in the past. Ted calmly said no thank you to the first offer, hung up, and between mouthfuls of sandwich, told me the Forrests' attorney would call back with a higher offer.

The sun streamed in through the wall of windows overlooking the city when the attorney called back with an additional increase that would cover the costs of the trial so far. Ted put him on hold and counseled me that if we asked for any more compensation, the case would likely be tied up in appeals for at least a year, and would be limited by the partial settlement agreement. Then Ted called his wife to ask her opinion, which I found very sweet. He next encouraged me to call Frank at home, to ask him for his thoughts. Frank's opinion was squarely to get the whole thing over with.

"I need one more opinion," I said to Ted after both of our spouses had sided with settling the case. I routed around in my wallet looking for a penny, while telling Ted and Mary Thomas' penny story.
In God We Trust.
"Heads we settle. Tails we finish the trial. Two out of three wins."
Heads.
Heads.
"We settle," I said.
And that was that.
Though my leg still hurt, I felt wonderfully lighter as we returned from lunch to the courtroom. We had avoided the mudslinging on the podium. No one had lost face, and the settlement was quite reasonable: particularly in light of the mystical experience, which I do not believe would ever have had a chance to come about without the accident. It was an integral part of the drama that took me apart, making space and reason for my shift in consciousness. For this, I would be forever grateful.

* * * * *

I was nearing the end of the yearlong requirement to be under evaluation by a psychiatrist (I'd settled on Dr. Greenbaum, who had given me yet a different diagnosis— post traumatic stress disorder— that I did not fit, as I didn't have the nightmares and flashbacks that are characteristic of this diagnosis). My compliance officer called to remind me that I needed to send in a formal request if I wanted the Investigative Committee to take any action on my behalf, to have the corrective action order terminated. He also recommended specific wording

Chapter 19: Loose Ends

in Dr. Greenbaum's report. But as I was unsuccessful in reaching Dr. Greenbaum to discuss these specifics with him, the thought came to me that perhaps a letter from Rabbi Avram would be equally sufficient to get the Board out of my life.

This would also give me the opportunity to work through the mystical experience with Avram. We'd never talked about it since my initial conversation with him, and I had felt a deep ache over our silence. I wanted to resolve the alienation I felt with him and with Judaism. I needed to know that there was a place within my spiritual tradition where what I had experienced could be accepted, valued, and supported. The message that I'd left Avram stated that I wanted to speak to him about a personal issue.

Avram was getting out of his car as I walked up to the building. My heart thumped madly and suddenly felt like a bag of stones.

"Hi," I smiled.

"Oh, hi. I'm just getting back from the Talmud class."

Avram's forehead sort of wrinkled with a look of surprise. He always looked so worried and serious around me since that day I shared my experience with him. But he relaxed a bit as we walked, and I talked about the wonderful rally for the plight of the homeless that he had helped organize the past weekend.

"I'm early, so if you need a couple of minutes I can wait," I said as he held the door for me and ushered me into the building.

"No, this is fine." We walked through the small foyer, past the secretary, and then stepped into his office. It is a nice-sized room, with a large desk and wonderful space for books on three of the walls. As I sat down in the chair in front of his desk, I noticed beautiful pictures of his wife and children in front of me. Rather than sitting with the desk between us, Avram sat down on a couch beneath his bookshelves and faced me from the other side.

I felt as though all the molecules between us were vibrating too fast and chaotically. My whole body was trembling in unison with the agitated rhythm.

Wanting to run away. I took a deep breath, and began to share the nature of my appointment with him.

"I'm a bit nervous," I began, legs crossed, arms trying to relax in my lap. "I was wondering if you would be able to write a letter on my behalf. It's related to the experience I had about two years ago, the one I spoke with you about. I don't know if you're aware of what's happened since then?"

"Why don't you fill me in," he answered, and leaned back, settling himself into the sofa.

I told him. I told him it all. About my boss, and the psychiatrists and the Board, and having my license suspended. I told him about what led up to the meditative experience: about things with Frank, the abortion the day before my accident, and my grief over it all for the next few months. Despite the time that had passed and the work I had done, my face twitched when I mentioned the abortion and I could feel the inner tension as I struggled to maintain my composure.

Avram tried to clarify that perhaps I wasn't grieving but depressed, that the word grief didn't touch what I had gone through. He was sympathetic about my experiences, but his understanding of the word depression was far different from my own clinical definition and its consequences. We never quite agreed on the word for my sadness, though it meant a lot to me. It was the difference between having a valid and healing emotional experience versus a pathological one. But I did not want to argue the issue again and decided to drop it and move on.

I took a deep breath and told Avram I was hoping for a letter for the Board stating that I'd been a stable, participating member of the congregation, and perhaps a statement about spiritual experiences not necessarily being an indication of some sort of mental pathology.

Chapter 19: Loose Ends

Avram laughed nervously and looked up. "That's *way* too general. What do you mean by "spiritual experience?" Looking at the stars and the ocean can be a spiritual experience. Reading Torah is a spiritual experience. Even making love can be a spiritual experience." He shook his head side-to-side. "And is there some problem practicing medicine with the diagnosis of bipolar disease?"

His words landed like a sledge hammer. I began to feel frantic inside again. "No," I managed to say calmly, "there's no problem practicing medicine with a diagnosis of bipolar disease, not as long as it's controlled. But I don't have a bipolar disorder."

His eyebrows arched higher. His eyes reflected the same look that Betsy had given me two years before when I'd said the same thing to her.

"What makes you think you don't?"

My skin began to crawl.

"Well, first of all, bipolar disease generally hits people in their twenties. It'd be quite uncommon for someone to get it out of the blue in their forties with no previous history of mental illness."

"Anything else?"

"Yes. Bipolar disease doesn't generally strike in the middle of meditating. Also, people with bipolar disease have trouble functioning because their inner reality is so different from our shared reality. In their manic phase, they can be so giving that they give away more than they have and can get in serious financial trouble. They can be so loving that they have problems with promiscuity. Marriages often fall apart from such excesses. None of this was an issue with me. On the contrary, my marriage was on the verge of falling apart before the mystical experience and the experience helped keep it together."

Avram went on to say that he knew many people with a diagnosis of bipolar disease who didn't show the excesses that I described.

I could feel my tension building into anger as I responded to Avram. "I personally believe that the labels of mania and hypomania are over diagnosed. I've worked with patients who were manic. Mania is a pathology. People who suffer from it can't function. They can't hold a conversation because their minds race so quickly they can't hold onto an idea. In my case, with the exception of philosophically tweaking the fears of my boss and the Board, I had no significant dysfunction. I was well aware of everything I was doing, even when I chose to approach my work in a lighter way. I'd just stepped into another state of consciousness and wasn't yet sure how much of the outer universe had followed me. But I had no problem acknowledging my error or communicating with others. I continued to manage the finances of my home, and met regularly with friends who had no concern over my mental status."

Avram continued to speak of people he knew who did not overtly express their disease, but who none-the-less took medication.

"What is it about them that needs medicating?" I asked.

He had a funny look on his face which inspired me to answer my own question. "Is it that they experienced things that most people didn't experience?"

Avram nodded with eyebrows arched.

"If I was alone in my experience, perhaps I'd think about taking medication too. But I'm not. What I experienced has been written about for thousands of years. It's a common experience in mystical traditions throughout the world and throughout all religions, though I'm not claiming to be a mystic. I'm just an ordinary person who had a mystical experience."

Avram still looked at me with disbelief.

"Have you ever heard of *Samadhi* ?" I asked, not knowing that within my own Hebrew language was a word of similar meaning, *Devekut*. The full union of self

Chapter 19: Loose Ends

with God.

"You think you had a Samadhi experience?" Again his eyebrows raised with a look of incredulity.

"Yes," I answered. "From all that I've read, what I experienced was just like that."

"Harriet, what you experienced wasn't real."

"But it was, Avram! It was very real! Not that this isn't real," I added, pointing to the room and its contents. "We experience different realities at the same time."

"I've heard those Beatles songs too."

"It's not a Beatles song!"

"I can see you're getting angry about this."

"You're right I'm angry! This isn't some fantasy I borrowed from the Beatles! Nor was it some fantasy that they created. You should understand these things! It's painful to have such a precious experience be thought of and spoken about as if it were a meaningless creation of my own, to have a personal experience of God that my religion has no place for, to be an outsider. It's incredibly alienating."

"I can imagine."

I sat back to take a breath, and in the pause, flashes of blessings came to mind.

"But it wasn't that bad. God was there all the time, and books and people were put in my path who validated what I experienced. Curiously, none of them were Jewish, except one woman who'd converted to Judaism from Catholicism and shares her identity with Sufism. She's become a good friend. Interestingly, she once had the diagnosis of bipolar disease *and* has had a mystical experience, and has talked with me about the difference."

I stared intently at the Rabbi, and continued with great difficulty, continued. "I was very hurt by your non-acceptance of what I experienced. I would have left the congregation and joined another synagogue, except that my kids wouldn't let me. They love you. And we love the people here and feel connected to everybody."

"Harriet, spiritual experiences aren't things that happen in a moment like that. You have to work up to them, work on them. It's how you live your life day by day."

How did he know how I lived my life? "I agree with you that how you live your life is a spiritual experience, probably the most important one. There isn't anything that isn't a spiritual experience, even when we are ignorant of that truth. AND there are experiences of expanded states of consciousness which can help to put the whole realm of spirituality and reality into a deeper and more useful context."

"Tell me, Harriet, do you want to return to this state of consciousness?"

I paused for a moment, looking at Avram. Dr. Eugene had asked me this same question at the end of my interview with him.

"I think it would be lovely to return to that experience, to return to such a pure and fearless state of being, of openness, of love. And it would be particularly wonderful if I could gather insights from such a state of mind that would allow me to be more effective in helping others. But it's not such an easy door to find again. It feels like my work is to practice focusing my thoughts, feelings, and actions so I can experience Oneness and Love as much as possible in my ordinary state of consciousness."

Then Avram asked me a question that came from nowhere I could understand. "Harriet, do you think that you've been wrong in any of this?"

"Wrong?" I paused. "That's a funny word, wrong. There are choices that I've made that I might not repeat. I have a deeper faith now. I've learned things along the way. But I don't think of any of this as wrong. All of it seemed necessary. I don't think anyone's been *wrong*. No one has intentionally tried to delude or harm anyone."

"Everybody who's been through something like this can usually find something they've done wrong."

He was leaning forward a little bit now, and I was

Chapter 19: Loose Ends

beginning to feel a little like Job.

"Well, I've got a laundry list of little things. Like just today, driving here, making a right turn while there was a pedestrian trying to cross who I didn't see because I wasn't paying enough attention and was in too much of a hurry."

Avram waved his hand and shook his head, "Psht. No, you know what I mean." He leaned forward again.

"Well, no. I don't think I've done anything wrong."

"Well, I think that's a problem. How can you have humility? How can you perform *teshuva* if you don't think you've done anything wrong?"

"You're allowed to think what you want to think, and I don't think you're wrong. But I resent you implying that I must have done something wrong."

I stood up calmly, not wanting him to see how upset I'd become, how quickly I wanted to get away from him. "I'm sorry this took so long. I went way over the fifteen minutes I thought it would take."

Avram nodded his head gently. "I figured it would take longer so I scheduled an hour."

"Thanks. And forget the letter."

He opened the door and it felt awkward having to walk by him in the doorway. I didn't reach out to shake hands or give him a hug. I tried to make it through the doorway keeping as far away from him as I could.

Frank came home shortly after I did and joined me in the kitchen, where I was fixing dinner. I didn't wait for him to forget to ask me how things went with Avram, but put my arms around him, and we gave each other a hug.

"Things with Avram were interesting," I began. "He doesn't seem to get it. Thinks I had a psychotic breakdown and seems to think that anyone who experiences something that others can't perceive needs to be on medication."

"So people in the past could have direct experiences with God, but not in the present," Frank responded thoughtfully.

"Yeah, it's too bad. I got so mad at him I even told him that his lack of acceptance of my experience for what it was almost made me leave the congregation. I can't believe I said that to him, but it's true. It's just so insensitive. And if it weren't for Iyra's Bat Mitzvah coming up, I probably would have left, too. She's so excited about it, so am I. And I don't dislike Avram. That's what makes this so hard. I respect him tremendously and value his wisdom and his efforts in the world. He's a passionately inspired man. I just don't understand where he's coming from on this issue.

"Mystical experiences are part of our humanity," I continued. "They move us beyond our old limited ways of being, into a bigger picture of Love and Connection. They teach us how to be in life in more deeply spiritual ways, more honest and more whole; and to truly feel the love for the other and the earth as ourselves. Our deepest wisdom, inspiration, and passion come from mystical experiences. And our capacity to have them is the only reason that I have any hope left for this world."

I took a deep breath and put my arms around Frank again. "Did I tell you recently that I love you? I love you even though it's not Valentine's Day any more, even though you didn't get me a card, or flowers, or anything once again."

"Well, that's good!" he smiled, and hugged me back sincerely.

"But try and remember next year. I like those things. And you have beautiful eyes. I've always thought it. But did I ever actually tell you that you have beautiful eyes?"

I was thinking today about some of the things Avram said, in particular, when he leaned forward and with all sincerity told me that what I experienced wasn't real. How completely opposite such an idea is

Chapter 19: Loose Ends

to Eastern ideologies which believe that life on earth is an illusion, Maya, and what is perceived in expanded states of consciousness is reality.

It's all reality.

Just as the pain we create by non-acceptance of other people's experiences and truths is also a reality.

Reality is the truth that one experiences.

But there are personal truths and collective truths, transient truths and eternal truths. Eternal truths can only be found at the crossroads where all religious teaching meets. Oneness and Love, Kindness, Compassion, the Wisdom to be discerning, Justice, Beauty, Balance, Honesty, Gratitude, Appreciation.

Justice. For every action, there is an opposite and equal reaction. This is justice.

Do unto others what you would have them do unto you. Justice.

Karma. The laws of life.

And what of Job? Somehow, I think Job still fits into this law. Unjust suffering must still be somehow in balance. Nature is nature. Maybe it's that balancing thing, where one person chooses to take on extra suffering to alleviate the suffering of others, while the world maintains its balance of joy and sorrow. Or maybe sometimes we just need a little cosmic inspiration to let go of a particular level of consciousness to keep evolving.

Karma? I wonder if we break the cycle of karma when we begin to see that which we despise in

Ghostwoman

others in ourselves and in our own history, and when we see in others the glory that we see in ourselves, and find joy in this way of seeing. Can we transcend some aspects of our duality by focusing on Love, the unified dimension of our reality?

The post office had some daphne blooming on the counter that the postman had forced open by bringing them inside. Inspired me to take the long way to the kitchen when I got home. With groceries in hand, I bypassed the front door and walked in sunlight along the cobbled path around the house. Lavender still blooms. I set my bags down to rub the blossoms in my hand and sniff. It is just as fragrant as the summertime.

The daffodil buds are getting taller each day and now the tulips and hyacinths are coming up, too. Looks like it's time to put out the slug bars; some of the tulips are getting chomped. The rhodie buds are looking very pregnant, and the perennials never died back completely this winter. That wispy blue thing that the hummingbirds liked is still alive, and it didn't even begin growing until July last year! And the Shasta daisy is still blooming; a new bud opened and a fresh flower is just beginning. The flowers that have been there since November are looking a little brown around the edges. But I cannot cut them. Flowers from Thanksgiving and Christmas should be allowed to gently fall away in their own time. They are miracles, and you just don't compost miracles.

Chapter 19: Loose Ends

Feb. 28, 2000

    Got a call from my compliance officer. Between Dr. Greenbaum's letter and my formal request, I've been redeemed! The investigative committee has signed off on me! Hallelujah!!!!!! Yeahhhhh!!!!

*   *   *   *   *

June, 2000

    Hours ago I was in Avram's office with Iyra, Sara, Eve and Laura, enjoying the discussion Avram led the girls through about their Torah portion. He did a wonderful job of asking questions, trying to probe some thoughtfulness out of their 13-year-old minds. He was kind, and not at all constricting about their interpretation of the piece. He didn't dictate his perspective but merely shared it, ending with the comment that Iyra and Sara were welcome to use any part of their conversation with him that might have moved them as they finish writing their drash, their personal interpretations and reflections on the story.

    Different days, different months, different roles. Bouncing off each other who we are, who we are becoming, ever changing; honing ourselves into who we choose to be, diving deep, deep down to get through difficult moments, that sometimes feel as if they will go on forever, but never do.

Ghostwoman

It's a syncopated life,
a half step off
from a perfect fit
IS
the rhythm that dances with Mystery.
The half step that is also a door, or a window,
to the light of Love
Creator of all
fills a ghostwoman with bones and blood, flesh,
and passion
to find the keys to her own happiness
and dance with
Life
is good.

Epilogue

Dr. Cohen continues to hold an active medical license, though her practice is limited to holistic therapy and energy medicine. She spent the previous year developing and leading a mindbody medicine skills group as well as a *Meditation is Medicine* group. She will be entering a Masters of Public Health program in the fall, with the desire to help integrate holistic healing philosophy and modalities into the public healthcare system, education and political systems.

She continues to be an active member in her old synagogue, studying Kabbalah with other like-minded individuals, and participating in social action and educational opportunities. She additionally feels great joy davening (praying) with congregation P'nai Or, and sharing their mystical interpretation and discussions of Torah

Harriet's greatest gift, challenge, and soul work continues to be to speak her truth. Gently, with compassion, and with right timing; but to speak it fully. She has discovered that truth likes to reside in a voice that expresses it, and when it is not honored, it can go into hiding. To change the world we must first change ourselves. Each truth, spoken compassionately, whittles away at the collective untruths, and brings us all closer to experiencing the eternal truth of our Oneness and our Love.

Ghostwoman

May our lives be expressions of our honesty, and our thoughts and actions, like tiny grains of sand, be our contributions to a more sustainable, loving, and beautiful world.

b'YaHaVaH.

Bibliography and Recommended Reading

1. *Anatomy of the Spirit* by Caroline Myss Ph.D.
2. *Wisdom of Healing* by David Simon, M.D.
3. *Path to Love* by Deepak Chopra
4. *Stalking Elijah* by Roger Kamenetz
5. *Many Lives, Many Masters* by Brian Weiss, M.D.
6. *The Book of Runes* by Ralph H Blum
7. *Spiritual Emergency* by Stanislav Grof
8. *They Say You're Crazy: How the worlds most powerful psychiatrists determine who is normal* by Paula Kaplan Ph.D.
9. *Are You Getting Enlightened or Losing Your Mind* by Dennis Gersten, MD
10. *Religions, Values, and Peak Experiences, and The Farther Reaches of Human Nature* by Abraham Maslow
11. *Toward a Psychology of Being* by Abraham Maslow
12. *Exceptional Human Experiences Journal* by Rhea White Ph.D.
13. *Healing Words* by Larry Dossey, MD
14. *The Essential Mystics, A Soul's Journey into Truth* by Andrew Harvey
15. *Remarkable Recovery* by Caryle Hirsch and Marc Ian Barasch

16. *Toxic Psychiatry* by Peter Breggin M.D.
17. *Women Who Run With the Wolves* by Clarissa Pinkola Estes Ph.D.
18. *God, Faith, and Health: Exploring The Spirituality-Healing Connection* Jeff Levine, Ph.D.

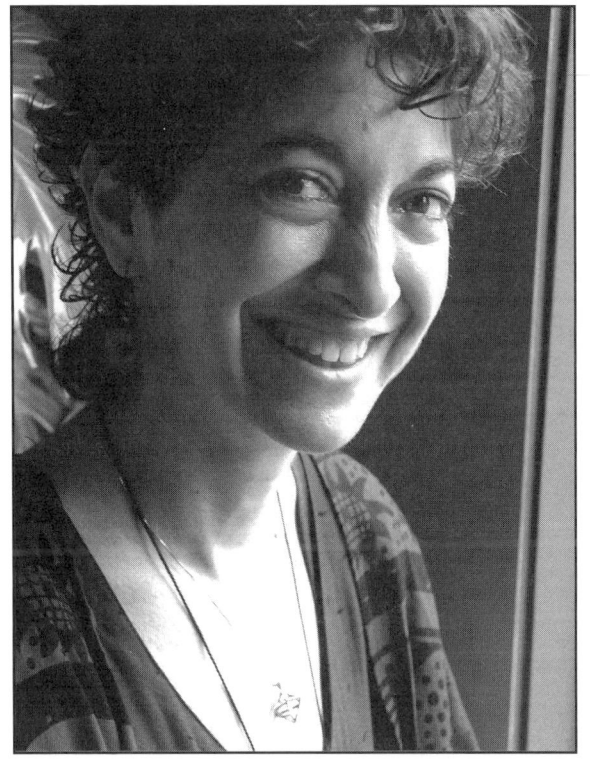

photo by Karen Downs

To order copies of *Ghostwoman,* or for information about meditation classes and energy medicine, Harriet can be reached at holisticooke@aol.com. Her website is pending.